Forsythe Natural Health GUIDE

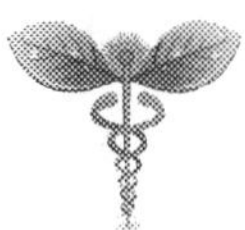

from A to Z

For Common Diseases and Symptoms

James W. Forsythe, M.D., H.M.D.

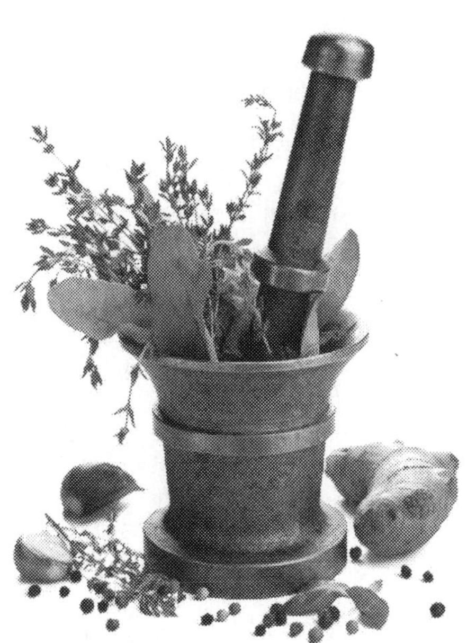

FORSYTHE NATURAL HEALTH GUIDE FROM A TO Z
For Common Diseases and Symptoms

Book Design: Patty Atcheson Melton

iUniverse books may be ordered through booksellers or by contacting:
iUniverse
1663 Liberty Drive
Bloomington, IN 47403
www.iuniverse.com
1-800-Authors (1-800-288-4677)

This book is a work of non-fiction. Unless otherwise noted, the author and the publisher make no explicit guarantees as to the accuracy of the information contained in this book and in some cases, names of people and places have been altered to protect their privacy.

The information, ideas, and suggestions in this book are not intended as a substitute for professional medical advice. Before following any suggestions contained in this book, you should consult your personal physician. Neither the author nor the publisher shall be liable or responsible for any loss or damage allegedly arising as a consequence of your use or application of any information or suggestions in this book.

Because of the dynamic nature of the Internet, any web addresses or links contained in this book may have changed since publication and may no longer be valid. The views expressed in this work are solely those of the author and do not necessarily reflect the views of the publisher, and the publisher hereby disclaims any responsibility for them.

ISBN: 978-1-4917-5239-5 (sc)
ISBN: 978-1-4917-5241-8 (hc)
ISBN: 978-1-4917-5240-1 (e)

Library of Congress Control Number: 2014919551

Print information is available on the last page.

iUniverse rev. date: 3/11/2015

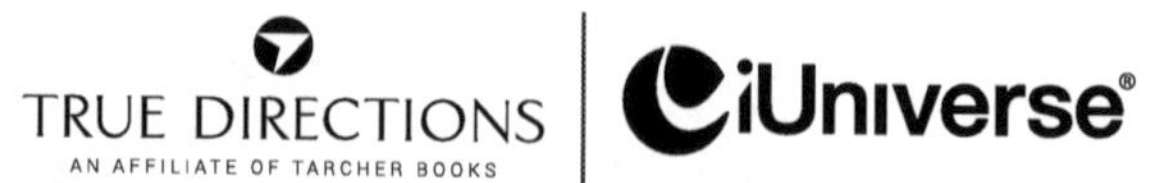

Dedication

To our Creator, who developed effective non-toxic natural remedies for almost every physical ailment known to mankind.

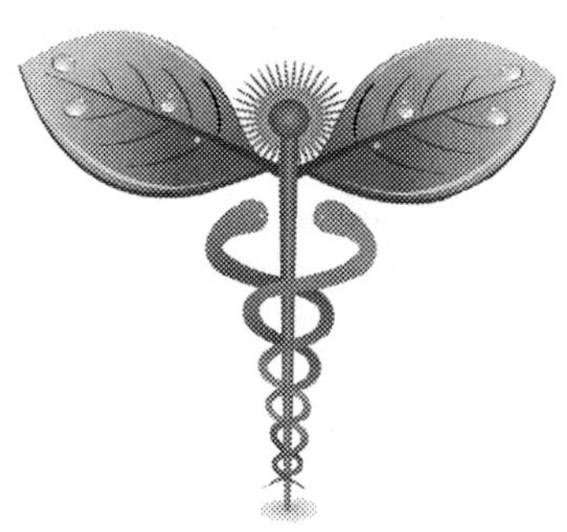

Contents

Introduction

Ultimately, all attempts to cure physical ailments hinges on a proper diet. The critical and often overlooked factor of optimal nutrition significantly helps prevent ailments, while also helping to correct health problems.

Every week people from around the world visit my health clinic, many of them asking what made them ill and the best ways to remedy the problems.

In most instances, I give this blunt answer: "Poor nutrition likely was a major contributor to your current ailment, and improved nutrition probably will help."

Of course, there are sometimes factors other than nutrition when considering likely causes, such as when a patient contracts a disease via sexual contact with another person, or injuries suffered from an accident. Yet even in these instances a lack of adequate nutrition can contribute to worsening symptoms when injured or exposed to sexually transmitted disease.

For the vast majority of ailments of all types, inadequate nutrition undoubtedly almost always has contributed to the problems—everything from cancer and heart disease to a wide variety of other ailments affecting vital organs such as the liver, pancreas and colon.

Thankfully, however, Mother Nature has blessed humanity with a miracle that comes in the form of natural foods—primarily crops and herbs that have been untainted by foreign substances.

Critical Factors Emerged

Sadly, on a worldwide basis many of the worst health problems suffered by the general public stem from inadequate nutrition.

Perhaps the worst culprits here are sugar, caffeine, processed meals, artificial preservatives and toxins that have dominated the United States' food supply.

Compounding these problems multi-fold, municipal water companies nationwide supply unsuspecting residents with harmful substances such as too much fluoride.

The heavy starches, sugars and toxins in the typical American diet lead to obesity, which has blossomed into the fastest-growing health epidemic in U.S. history.

Many scientists worry that the death rate from obesity and overweight issues will skyrocket during the early and mid-21st Century.

The problem seems particularly bothersome when taking into account the fact that many of the most dangerous foods in the American diet are actually addictive.

Why These Problems Exist

Far more pervasive and deadly than many of us realize, today's U.S. food manufacturers strive to make food as palatable as possible. Essentially, this means that to the person eating these foods, the meals or snacks have a yummy, extremely satisfying taste found nowhere in nature.

Food manufacturers perform this "trickery" by overloading today's foods with sugar—perhaps one of the biggest culprits in sparking overweight and obesity issues. Over many thousands or perhaps millions of years, the human body never had to process white sugars.

The onset of vastly improved farming and shipping techniques enabled industry to start supplying consumers with dangerous sugars starting in the 1700s. By the late 1800s sugar had become a mainstay of the typical American diet.

Another major offender is starchy foods, which generally come in the form of pizzas, donuts, muffins, tarts and pie crusts.

Normally, when eaten infrequently these substances would not necessarily pose a huge problem for individual people. However, judging from a variety of studies and my personal observations, people unknowingly become addicted to these harmful foods while eating them in dangerously excessive quantities.

The extremely high level of palatability makes these substances seemingly irresistible to a disturbingly high percentage of Americans—most who fail to realize they're "actually addicted" to these foods.

We Feed Ourselves Poison

Whether or not people want to hear this, as an overall sector of the world's population American society is literally poisoning itself to death with bad food.

Quite disturbingly without necessarily realizing that this is happening, consumers have unwittingly allowed themselves to "become victims" of the food industry.

Determined to boost profit, food companies manufacturing meals on an industrial scale have loaded foods with excess levels of artificial preservatives.

This is intended to make food easy to quickly process and to store for as long as possible, while getting products onto store shelves lightning-fast.

Some of the worst selections are frozen meals for cooking in ovens or via microwave. An added danger emerges when manufacturers instantly wrap foods in plastics and aluminum, which contain metals and toxins harmful to the body.

When eaten consistently over extended periods, people who consume these foods often suffer from a buildup of dangerous, life-threatening toxins in their bodies due to food contaminated by packaging.

The Vicious Treadmill Keeps Turning

Unknowingly and unwittingly, Americans of all ages have essentially become proverbial rats stuck on treadmills upon which they're force-fed unhealthy foods.

The addictive and overly palatable characteristics of these foods mask the toxins, sugars and artificial preservatives that steadily ravage critical organs.

Some of the worst of these initially unseen symptoms begin in childhood, the teens or young adult years—only to steadily harm vital bodily functions over time.

One of the typical early "victims" in this process is the liver. When healthy that organ removes toxins, excess fat and other invaders from the blood. This is so critical that without a healthy liver a person would suffer liver damage.

The danger worsens even further when harmful bacteria, "bad cholesterol," and caffeine damage the intestines, circulatory system and adrenal functions.

People Make Poor Meal Choices

Besides the dangers imposed by food producers, far too many people are making bad or negative food choices for themselves and for their families.

Either recklessly or unknowingly, consumers buy and consume far too many harmful fats, high-sugar candy, alcoholic beverages and dangerous over-the-counter remedies.

These foods, beverages and substances clog arteries, destroy liver function, generate excess belly fat and destroy or hinder the functioning of various essential organs.

When these foods are eaten consistently over time the person typically becomes steadily hungry as their bodies desperately crave adequate nutrients.

Yet the cascading, steadily increasing damage works as a proverbial "domino effect," coupled with palatability. This leads the person to continually eat far too much of the very foods that are steadily damaging his overall health.

Poor-Quality Crops Prevail

As if the dangerous additives and poor food choices weren't already enough to cause major concern, many crops today contain less nutrients than in the past.

Some scientists fear that over-farming or growing crops on the same plots of land consistently over time has seriously depleted soils. This situation, in turn, can lead to pernicious conditions where crops lack vital minerals and inadequate amounts of critical vitamins people need to thrive and to remain healthy.

The situation worsens multi-fold when taking into account the fact that increasing numbers of food manufacturers are growing and distributing "genetically modified crops." This means that scientists intentionally modify the DNA within these crops, all in a dangerous effort to boost farming productivity and ultimately profitability.

Many people fear that such foods—typically called genetically modified organisms or GMOs—are irreversibly damaging the critical, essential DNA of people who eat them.

If true, as some studies seem to suggest, people suffering from the ravages of DNA modification pass those harmful characteristics on to their children. The resulting symptoms might include physical deformities, inadequate organ function or the development of extremely serious or life-threatening health problems.

Corrupt Politicians and Corporations Created the Problem

Dastardly, self-serving and selfish politicians, huge food corporations and U.S. government agencies work together to perpetuate and to exacerbate the problem.

Tens of thousands of political lobbyists work on Capitol Hill to aggressively protect and to push forward with their own best interests—"the public health be damned."

As a result, the overall governmental regulations and oversight of the farming industry and the pharmaceutical business has been lax and poorly managed.

The U.S. Food and Drug Administration, commonly known as the "FDA," is among the worst offenders. The regulators at this gargantuan federal agency are overly influenced by today's food manufacturers and particularly by the big drug companies.

Sometimes called "Big Pharma," the devilish huge drug

companies want to convince the general public that nutrients, vitamins and minerals are actually harmful to health.

Ultimately, the drug companies want the public to avoid natural, effective vitamins, minerals and herbs, instead taking extremely dangerous and harmful drugs that seriously threaten overall health. Big Pharma wants us to believe that natural substances are harmful, while from the huge drug companies view "only drugs should be used to cure ailments."

The Media Also Threatens Public Health

As an overall sector, the reckless and lazy U.S. news media has perpetuated this problem. Some of the worst damage occurred in the last few months of 2013, when the FDA announced that vitamins and supplements are ineffective while also dangerous to public health.

Either lazy or too understaffed to look deeply into this matter, the vast majority of media outlets simply reprinted or rebroadcast the FDA statements almost verbatim.

The sad fact was that the public was never told the truth, namely that vitamins and minerals are essential to good health while preventing diseases. As God intended, Mother Nature has provided the best, most effective and efficient non-toxic remedies for a vast array of ailments, diseases and adverse physical conditions.

Ultimately, everything at the heart of these corporate, governmental and political issues comes down to one thing and to one word—"money."

You see, as previously stated, Big Pharma wants to boost profits to maximum levels. Such firms cringe at the thought that people can benefit from effective, low-cost natural remedies

This is why if Big Pharma had its way, the corrupt FDA bureaucrats pushing to fulfill the objective of major drug companies would outlaw Vitamin C and any of a vast array of other beneficial natural substances.

Typical Diet Selections Impose Dangers

As if these factors weren't already enough to rise concerns, many seemingly healthy selections within typical American diet selections impose extreme dangers to public health.

Perhaps the most potentially catastrophic of these is sodium or salt, loaded at severely high quantities in numerous foods—particularly potato chips and crackers.

A typical American eats far too much salt yearly, a particular threat to maturing people due to the propensity of high blood pressure caused by too much sodium.

While loading the liver with far too many toxicants and chores, excessive salt often makes a person feel a continually unquenched thirst. Meantime, the high blood pressure leads to heart disease or even stroke, severe conditions that can cause death.

Needless to say, a person might feel overwhelmed, confused and even depressed when faced with this potentially catastrophic labyrinth of serious dangers from all these various foods, additives, preservatives, sugars.

Yet as a physician now entering my fifth decade of practice I now feel a burning need to teach the public about a vast array of healthful options and remedies. These are made possible by Mother Nature, in the form of beneficial foods, minerals and vitamins.

History Proves the Effectiveness of Natural Foods

Until the mid-1990s I practiced solely as an oncologist treating cancer patients with poisonous chemotherapy as mandated by standard protocol imposed by that profession.

For the first 20 years of my practice beginning in the mid-1970s the survival rate of my Stage IV cancer patients mirrored the dismal national statistics of about 2 percent at the five-year mark.

"There has to be a better way," I told myself, finally deciding in the mid-1990s to study for a degree needed to practice as a licensed homeopath capable of administering, recommending or prescribing natural remedies.

As a result, I became one of only a handful of integrative

medical oncologists practicing in the United States. Since then, incorporating natural remedies into treatments, the survival rate of my Stage IV cancer patients reached more than 60 percent at the four-year mark

Along the way, I also began administering or prescribing various natural remedies for patients suffering from a wide variety of non-cancerous ailments. Much of the time these efforts have been successful, incorporating natural foods and herbs into the lifestyle of patients—enabling many of them to recover from a variety of health issues, while regaining good health.

The Public Needs to Know These Cures

Bowing to demand from patients and other homeopaths worldwide, in 2013 I issued one of the more than 14 books I have written—the "Forsythe Anti-Cancer Diet." That publication remains a steady, strong seller in international markets in both "paper-book" form and as an eBook.

The steady and intense public demand for the critical information on how healthy foods and herbs help our bodies motivated me to write the book you're reading now.

Besides cancer patients and people striving to avoid that disease, consumers worldwide are beginning to realize that they're essentially being force-fed poisons and propaganda by the food industry, Big Pharma and lazy politicians.

Eager to bring the truth to the public, I took the time and effort needed to carefully analyze many of the most common physical ailments. Listed in alphabetical order here alphabetically from A to Z, these many ailments virtually all have non-toxic, natural remedies provided by Mother Nature.

I imagine that until getting this publication many people have never heard of these many natural remedies, let alone the horrific dangers imposed by today's food and pharmaceutical industries.

Take Positive Action with This Information

Essentially in the many pages that follow I've armed the general public with the "truth" that they need to avoid and to treat a vast array of ailments and adverse health conditions that range from minor to severe.

For the majority of these ailments I strongly recommend that you use these natural remedies under the guidance of a licensed homeopath or a professional practitioner of natural medicines—such as a professional in Naturopathy, or an integrative family practitioner

Although generally unknown by the American public, many of these effective natural remedies have been used in other cultures for hundreds or thousands of years.

Steadily over time spanning thousands of years these specific plant-based herbal remedies emerged in diverse environmental conditions worldwide.

Numerous cultures found and identified a vast majority of these remedies, many that work amazingly well—far better, in fact, in many instances than dangerous, toxic, addictive and expensive drugs pushed by Big Pharma.

Legal, Harmless and Effective Remedies

Everything comes down to the fact that today's giant companies "don't want you to know about these effective remedies."

It's true.

In fact, if Big Pharma and Big Food had their way the book that you're reading now never would have reached the marketplace.

As previously stated, everything comes down to money. Natural remedies such as herbs and natural whole foods are far less expensive than drugs. Just as impressive, lots of the time people don't need to pay a doctor for examinations, in order to eventually receive expensive prescriptions.

An added benefit emerges from the fact that most natural remedies work on the underlying causes of illness, rather than merely masking symptoms like Big Pharma does.

While temporarily blocking symptoms, many Big Pharma products enable or allow the underlying causes of poor health to perpetuate and to worsen.

This serves as yet another reason why whenever possible today's consumers should avoid standard allopathic physicians who only are allowed to prescribe Big Pharma drugs, never recommending natural remedies.

Many consumers lucky enough to know the truths that I've set forth here cringe at the dogma embraced by standard doctors trained to tell patients that natural substances are "useless quackery from snake-oil salesmen."

Take Advantage of Mother Nature

Armed with the basics found within this introduction, you should feel free to browse through or to thoroughly read the remainder of this book.

What you'll soon discover is the good news that, yes indeed, natural remedies and prevention measures exist for almost every typical ailment and disease.

For patients striving to benefit from natural medicines, as previously stated success will hinge on a healthy diet coupled with herbs and various natural plant-based substances.

Many of these herbs are found at relatively low cost in drugstores, supermarkets and from sellers specializing in herbs, vitamins, minerals and supplements.

A good start often entails a visit to and an examination by a licensed homeopath. As consistently stated in many of my other books, consumers should strive to refrain from attempting to diagnose themselves—especially when severe ailments are involved.

Give Yourself Thanks

Many patients and consumers worldwide say they "cannot possibly thank me enough" for providing this information.

Yet more importantly I prefer to stress the fact that people eager to benefit from a natural and effective health maintenance and healing strategy should instead thank themselves for taking this vital quest.

An age-old saying tells us that "information is power." Indeed, with this vital and easy-to-understand data consumers can empower themselves to achieve improved health, while also avoiding the many pitfalls imposed by the typical American diet.

Sure enough, thanks to the essential information that follows in many instances you and your loved ones can easily over time benefit from a natural pathway to good health.

-James W. Forsythe, M.D., H.M.D.

A

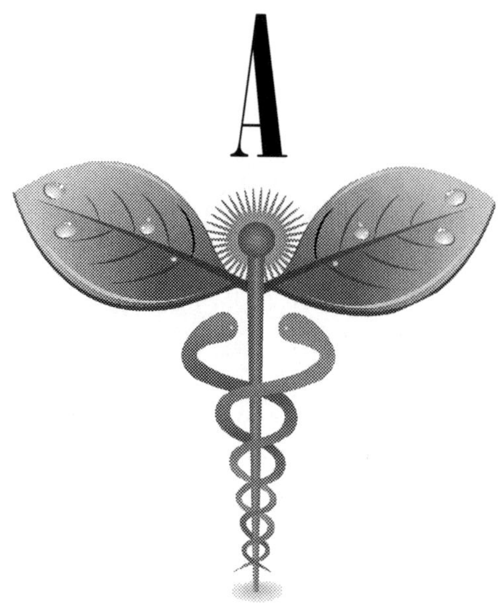

Acne

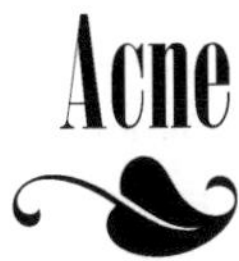

Pimples

This adverse skin condition can occur at any time during life, particularly puberty as many of the body's various hormones begin to click into gear. The development of acne signals that one or more processes within the body have gone off kilter. Everyone suffering from acne, particularly teenagers should strive to avoid feeling embarrassed because doing so causes stress—a frequent cause of this condition.

Acne Causes

The body increases its cell production during puberty, often triggering acne which initially forms within the skin's follicles. The various bodily changes that teens undergo during this stage of life often mix or combine in generating pimples. The body's new increased production of testosterone circulates to various parts of the body, particularly the face—the greatest area of concern. Interestingly, not everyone suffers acne during their teens or other life stages. Each person's skin and particularly the pores react in varying ways to this increase in oil. Some people experience excessive or unsightly skin growths or eruptions in regions where the openings of oil ducts get covered or clogged. The situation worsens in instances where growing or spreading acne accelerates skin cell production, thereby oiling and clogging additional skin pores. Among specific causes:

Sugars: Eating foods high in sugars generates bacteria overgrowth, while also making the blood overly acidic. Similar or related problems sometime erupt from menstrual cycles in women, excessive stress, adverse reactions to drugs and constipation that gradually or suddenly builds up due to foreign or unneeded substances within the body.

Allergies: A wide variety of food and inhalent allergies.

Substances: Any oil, cream or make-up intentionally or inadvertently put on the face can irritate the skin—increasing the probability of acne infections or clogged pores.

Dirty skin: Failing to clean or to adequately wash the skin can worsen blackheads and whiteheads. Deficiencies in various substances such as B vitamins, Vitamin A or magnesium sometimes naturally rob the body of its ability to fight acne.

Toxins: When a person fails to have regular, predictable and healthy bowel movements, various toxins build up within the body before being eliminated through the pores. This unwanted process irritates the skin, which becomes vulnerable to acne infection. Certain chemo agents, particularly "targeted agents," stimulate acne.

Acne Treatments

Throughout history, doctors, families and various cultures have used or developed various remedies or lifestyle changes to clear the skin or treat acne. Among essentials:

Increase: Drink lots of water and eat plenty of watermelon and raw foods. Add Vitamin C and B-complex vitamins.

Stress: Reduce or eliminate stress. (See the "stress" section of this guide for tips on this.)

Foods: Stop eating or lessen the consumption of foods considered as "acne triggers," particularly sugars, dairy, meats, processed food, fried foods and soft drinks.

Avoid Touching

Avoid touching your acne because doing so actually worsens the condition, when bacteria and oils from your fingers cause the condition to spread or to become infected. So, when and if you must squeeze a pimple, sterilize your hands and fingers by washing, ideally with alcohol-based bacterial gel, or hire a professional to handle this chore. Additionally, teen boys and young men should avoid razor shaving when suffering acne.

Skin cleansing

Besides controlling diet and beverages, a key to eliminating and preventing acne is to keep the skin clean of excess oils. Use mild soap before rinsing with hydrogen peroxide. Afterward, let the skin dry before washing again with clean water. Then, lightly spray the face with "Willard Water." To remove impurities, use clay to cover the face, letting the mixture dry before washing away—thereby removing impurities.

Bodily Mechanisms

The key to controlling or preventing acne entails preventing the buildup of fast-forming skin cells that clog pores with oils. An initial strategy involves avoiding foods high in fatty acids, animal fats and refined carbohydrates.

A primary goal strives to prevent the blood from becoming too acidic, a condition considered the primary cause of acne by many health experts. While eliminating these potentially harmful foods, take these steps to heal or eliminate acne.

Water: Drink plenty of pure, clean water daily. Some health experts deem water as the "universal solvent," recommending that everyone—particularly those suffering from acne—drink at least eight 12-ounce glasses daily. Watermelon juice also improves the skin's health and overall appearance.

Vitamins: Along with specific minerals, certain vitamins at specific amounts can work wonders in fortifying the skin with a healthy glow. A great starter often involves Vitamin C at 3 to 5 grams daily, plus Vitamin A (10,000 IU) in tablet form or as a beta-carotene from natural foods. (Important: Pregnant women or those who could become pregnant should avoid excessive amounts of Vitamin A. Such individuals should consult their physicians.)

Fibers: Eat plenty of fiber-rich foods, particularly vegetables that can be cooked or more preferably raw. Enjoy vegetables as snacks rather than sugars or fatty acids. Other great fiber sources include whole-grain bread, brown rice and legumes. Such foods fortify and clean the digestive tract, often leading to a healthy overall body and clear skin.

ADD / ADHD

Attention Deficit Disorder (ADD) / Attention Deficit Hyperactivity Disorder (ADHD) / Developmental Coordination Disease (DCD)

While almost every child occasionally becomes rowdy, when such behavior becomes excessive in an individual youngster the condition can curtail the ability to learn—while also hindering the ability to "cope" with life. Children experiencing such systems are sometimes diagnosed with ADD or attention deficit disorder, or ADHD, attention deficit hyperactivity disorder.

According to various published reports, some researchers believe a least 12 percent of children under age 16 suffer from this condition—a medical condition that some health experts believe is increasing. Worsening matters, at least by some estimates, a whopping 60 percent of children with ADHD still have such symptoms upon becoming adults. Among common behaviors considered as symptoms:

Outbursts: Angry tirades characterized by disruptive or defiant behavior

Learning problems: The rowdy behavior hampers the ability to concentrate for extended periods

Sudden unpredictable behavior: An inability to—or an extreme difficulty in—controlling reactions

Hyperactive: Unable to become calm; restlessness

ADD / ADHD Causes

The condition is considered a disorder of the body's nervous and emotional system. Much of the time this entails problems with the person's "neuro developmental," a process that in healthy people results in the generating, shaping and reshaping of the nervous system. Various medical professionals and scientists disagree on the causes and potential treatments. Much of the blame usually focuses on "poor nutrition." Adding to the issue, some practitioners of natural treatments cite what they consider "dysfunctional environments," everywhere from the home, church or school. Although medical professionals have disagreement on this overall issue, some commonly accepted theories have emerged. Among them:

Toxicity: Toxic mercury derived from vaccines, or dental amalgams

Nutrition: A lack of adequate nutrition, combined with an excess of sugar or high-glucose foods

Environment: Exposure to toxins while in the womb or during early childhood, especially drugs and alcohol

Trauma: Apparent brain injury in the womb, during childbirth or early childhood

Inherited traits: A "genetic predisposition" to such behaviors or symptoms, especially bipolar disorder

ADD / ADHD Treatments

A majority of health professionals seem to claim that there is "no cure." Thus, their goal is to keep the symptoms or adverse behaviors "in check," thereby striving to optimize cognitive functioning. Various health experts disagree on this overall conclusion, issuing differing opinions on the precise definition of these conditions. Meantime, some experts argue that natural remedies offer a good chance of "curing" or managing the condition. Although universal agreement remains lacking, many experts recommend that treatments be combined in nutritional, psychological and cognitive combinations that include:

Stress: Strive to reduce, minimize or eliminate stress via relaxation and calming techniques. (See the section on Stress)

Dysfunction: Reduce ineffective communication and personal interaction at home by having the entire family visit mental health or social experts

Overall diet: Avoid eating foods that contain suspected

allergens or toxins, and instead eat an "antioxidant rich" diet that contains sufficient Vitamin C and Vitamin E supplements.

Foods: Eat natural selections ranging from bee pollen, kelp, and green leafy vegetables to Spirulina dietary supplement, while ignoring sugary, fatty foods such as candy, cheese, candy, soda and fried meals.

Avoidance: Steer clear of food additives suspected as allergens, ranging from processed meats and dairy products to wheat.

Bolster: Increase ingestion of omega fatty acids, either through foods or supplements.

Unique Feature

Numerous experts insist that herbs, particularly at least 500 milligrams of daily magnesium, can generate calming sensations while relieving symptoms. Some children balk at attempts to avoid sugary junk food. So, consider taking the family on what health experts call a "good-foods vacation," away from tempting but harmful treats.

Adrenal Imbalance

Adrenal Depletion / Adrenal Fatigue / Burnout

The body's vital and essential adrenal glands can literally suffer from what scientists call "adrenal exhaustion" when overused. One of the most common afflictions here is called "chronic fatigue syndrome." The overall condition of adrenal imbalance has been cited for a wide variety of maladies. These range from heart disease and blood sugar imbalances to off-kilter hormone levels, imbalanced blood sugar, inefficient digestion and an inconsistent or inefficient overall metabolism.

A wide variety of factors can cause or trigger adrenal exhaustion. These range from a variety of viruses including Epstein-Barr virus, and herpes virus 6, plus stress or an excessive use of stimulants like caffeine. The problem is so severe that drinking too much caffeine or artificial stimulants can ultimately exhaust the adrenal system.

When initially drinking too much caffeine or ingesting other potentially harmful stimulants your energy levels might temporarily accelerate. At the start this might generate a healthful sensation of being "wired" or "speedy." Yet such symptoms might actually serve as a clear indicator that your adrenal glands are generating too much adrenaline. This factor, in turn, might result in trouble concentrating while losing appetite. These conditions leave the adrenal glands exhausted, generating varying symptoms as cortisol disappears within the body. Among them:

Decreased sex drive

Back pain

Light-headed sensations due to low blood pressure

Decreased blood sugar

Sleepiness with poor-quality sleep

Tender lymph notes

Continual fatigue no matter how much sleep

Insufficient energy for everyday activities

Other negative symptoms might include moodiness, headaches, low appetite and irregular sleep patterns.

Adrenal Imbalance Causes

Physicians and scientists list a wide range of likely overall causes for adrenal imbalance, which is actually by definition a "hormone imbalance." Within healthy people the adrenal glands pump out numerous hormones essential for vital energy needed in order to maintain life, enabling the person to flee or to fight if necessary to survive. Yet these "fight or flight" mechanisms go off kilter when the adrenal glands fail to generate vital cortisol, which helps healthy people cope with stress and fear. Added complexity comes into play when considering the fact that these hormones impact chemicals impacting the body's vital functions—everything from blood sugar to the regulation of magnesium, sodium and potassium. When one or more functions go awry as a result of adrenal imbalances, a negative chain reaction can erupt. Among common causes:

Inadequate sleep
Excessive caffeine
Food allergies, including sensitivity to gluten and wheat
Artificial stimulants
Digestive problems

Adrenal Imbalance Treatments

Right away people suffering from adrenal imbalances need to change their lifestyles. Their adverse physical conditions usually are the result of poor or inadequate lifestyle choices or habits, everything from the foods they eat to a lack of stress relievers. Among the key choices in order to reverse the problems:

Stimulants: Reduce the consumption of caffeine or other artificial stimulants, avoiding coffee or sodas and other beverages containing artificial stimulants.

Stress reduction: Cut down on stress within the mind and body by making lifestyle changes, meditating, and exercise. (See the section on Stress)

Supplements: Take a steady regimen of minerals and vitamins, including magnesium and potassium, and Pantothenic acid plus vitamins B, C and E.

Natural: Ingest organic maca root derived from super-food supplements

Foods: Avoid foods that contain toxins, and increase protein-rich foods while decreasing carbohydrates and sugars.

Allergies

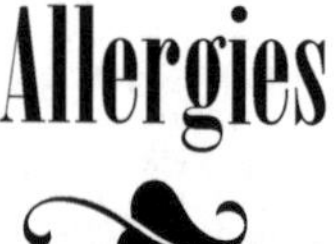

Also see the sections on Liver and Gallbladder Health, Immune System Health, Candida, Hives, Bee Stings and Insect Bites

One of the human body's most formidable mechanisms involves the immune system, which enables people to biologically battle potentially troublesome biological invaders.

Yet extreme trouble and even a danger of death erupts when the body's immune system goes into overdrive—doing far too much to ward off foreign substances. Such a condition is commonly called an "allergy."

Invaders that can trigger allergies enter the body via ingestion, by inhaling the substances through the air, or even by coming into physical contact with the allergen in a condition that scientists call "hypersensitivity." Compounding the problem, a wide variety of common allergens exist. These range from mold, dust and dander to pollen, synthetic chemicals and foods.

When an individual person is allergic to one of these substances, upon contact the body's various immune systems click into overdrive. These "allergic reactions" result in everything from excessive mucus to itching, sneezing, teary eyes and coughing or congestion. Some of the worst reactions that emerge into potentially life-threatening conditions can include extreme difficulty breathing and massive inflammation.

Allergy Causes

The immune system becomes imbalanced, generating "allergy symptoms." The causes of these imbalances result from excessive toxins within the body, deficiencies or over-saturation of certain foods or nutritional levels that go off kilter.

Additional Considerations

Allergy systems are often best treated or prevented naturally, rather than using synthetic and potentially dangerous prescription pharmaceuticals. Among suggested natural remedies: grape seed extract and rosemary essential oil as anti-inflammatory treatments; the marshmallow root herb for reducing mucus; stinging nettle for hay fever; and burdock root in tincture, tea, pine oil essential oil congestion and bee pollen.

Allergy Treatments

Drink water: One of the most formidable weapons to combat or prevent allergies involves drinking lots of clean water on a continual, regular and daily basis.

Natural: To strengthen the immune system, ingest lots of natural substances and vitamins, particularly vitamins A, C and E plus Echinacea and goldenseal.

Toxicity: Avoid toxic substances, particularly by ending long-term prescription medications.

Avoidance: Stay away from and refuse to eat foods most frequently identified as "common allergens," such as wheat or dairy.

Cleanse: Clean your organs, particularly the liver and intestines, by eating lots of foods and herbs such as milk thistle and apple juice known to help address this problem.

These various tactics can become formidable, largely because liver malfunctions play a significant role in contributing to allergies. Also, avoiding dairy products can become significant, since such foods can contribute to upper-respiratory allergies like asthma and hay fever. Some people have benefited from miraculous treatments for airborne allergies thanks to raw bee pollen—which must be kept frozen. To help rebuild or fortify the adrenal glands ingest 2 grams of Vitamin C with food in the morning and at bedtime along with 150 milligrams of adrenal cortex extract and 1 gram of pantothenic acid.

Alzheimer's Disease

Senile Dementia, Also, Alzheimer's type [SDAT]

The loss of memory commonly associated with Alzheimer's Disease is often associated with "old age," a form that health professionals call "senile dementia." Sadly, various researchers have estimated that about half of people over age 85 suffer from this condition, while one tenth of individuals age 65 or older suffer from the condition. To varying degrees or levels in individual patients brain function deteriorates, adversely impacting emotional and intellectual functioning. Besides memory loss, a major concern sometimes emerges as the brain physically deteriorates.

Compounding these problems, some people with Alzheimer's Disease become paranoid, overly aggressive, disoriented, depressed or physically fatigued. Among common symptoms are: a disoriented sense of time; problems speaking fluently; the loss of short- or long-term memory; and problems understanding numbers.

Alzheimer's Disease Causes

A wide variety of potential triggers have been identified, although scientists admit they still fail to fully understand the condition. Among the likely causes are genetics or hereditary conditions; poor pH balances within the body; a toxic buildup of heavy metals; hormonal imbalances; and nutritional deficiencies in substances vital to optimal brain function—such as magnesium, folic acid, niacin from Vitamin B3; tryptopahan; zinc; and vitamins B6, B12; C, D and E.

Additional Considerations

Some researchers blame the onset of a percentage of Alzheimer's cases on a decline in the essential fatty acid prosphatidyserine, a condition that sometimes progresses with age. Foods that increase the brain's energy and maintain oxygen-rich blood such as Coenzyme Q10 also have been listed as a potential way to lessen Alzheimer's symptoms or to delay progression of the disease. In some studies Alzheimer's patients have experienced increases in memory and attention spans after taking Chinese Ginkgo biloba tree herbal extracts.

Alzheimer's Disease Treatments

Scientists and medical professionals have developed a variety of treatments often deemed effective at least to some degree—although there remains no "cure" for the condition. People with blood relatives who currently suffer from or who have had Alzheimer's face a greater likelihood of getting the condition. Among recommended preventative measures:

Exercise: Increases blood flow throughout the body, and particularly the brain.

Tension: Reduce stress via exercise, yoga, saunas and techniques. (See the section on Stress)

Amino acids: Eat high-protein foods or substances loaded with anti-oxidants.

Games: Engage in lots of brain games or puzzles, or even learn a different language. People who learn a different language after age 60 cut their Alzheimer's risk by half, according to some studies. Playing or remembering music is the last to go.

Meals: Eating lots foods such as spinach, alfalfa and garlic that cause chelating are often considered effective.

Supplements: Anti-inflammatory supplements like curry, and cayenne can prove formidable along with vitamins B, C and E.

Anxiety

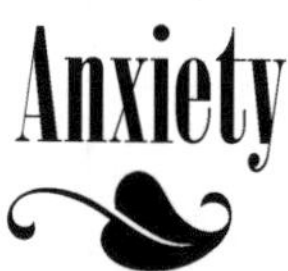

Anxiety Disorder / Panic Attack, Also see the Stress section

At various times in life just about everyone feels at least some anxiety under specific conditions, such as when having to sing, talk or play-act in front of other people. Sometimes anxiety occurs for no specific reason without causing major problems before subsiding or disappearing. Sadly, however, for some people anxiety occurs regularly, causing dangerous or potentially debilitating symptoms. These range from disorientation, pale skin, shaking and dizziness to excessive sweating and heart palpitations. Full-blown anxiety attacks can disrupt the person's life, disturbing sleep, generating moodiness and sparking disorders within the body's nervous system.

Physicians sometimes diagnose "anxiety disorder" when such symptoms disrupt the person's normal or otherwise healthy life.

Anxiety Causes

Researchers from a variety of medical specialties often pinpoint the "cause" of anxiety as the patient's sense of foreboding or fear—even in instances where the individual should have no "logical reason" to feel that way. Stored-up internal emotions within the person build up, before suddenly erupting due to certain life events that trigger panic attacks and anxiety. This often results in excessive stress as the individual strives to release the psychological, emotional and physical buildup of fear and anxiety.

Anxiety Treatments

The best natural and most effective treatment are to identify the underlying problem or emotional factors that trigger the condition. This sometimes becomes challenging. Success here hinges on the patient's willingness to strive to target emotional issues, coupled with what type of method a medical professional uses. Among strategies that some physicians and homeopaths have deemed helpful or effective:

Supplements: Take healthful quantities of kava and Saint John's wort, famous for calming and depression-blocking qualities.

Sugars: Reduce or eliminate sugary foods, plus carbohydrates.

Proteins: Eat more high-protein foods, while also ingesting "super food" to boost the body's overall intake of healthy nutrients.

Avoid: Never ingest caffeine and diet pills while also eliminating stress.

Soothing foods: Ingest more foods and herbs packed with "calming" attributes, such as valerian root, chamomile, passion fruit and passionflower.

Techniques: Using "emotional clearing" methods such as psychotherapy is sometimes effective. Other lesser-known strategies also have sometimes been effective, such as Neuro-Emotional Technique (NET) and Neuro Linguistic Programming (NLP).

Management: To manage, lessen or prevent panic attacks as they're starting or occurring, keep plenty of grounding and calming essential oils with you. These can include myrrh, lavender oil, cedar wood and spruce oil.

Alternative strategies: Seldom-used or little-known methods sometimes are effective such as laughing, meditating and yoga, or striving to control the breathing process. Massages help.

Exercise: Moving the body vigorously generates the internal natural production of dopamine and serotonin, which relive anxiety within the brain and make people "feel good." A peculiar trait of patients with this dementia is their continued ability to recognize and to play music.

Arthritis

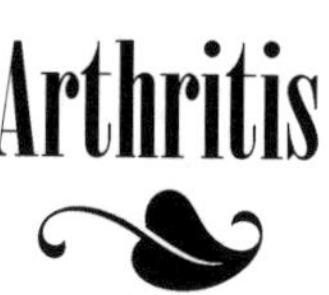

Joint Pain

Also visit sections on Inflammation, Infection, Bursitis

Many patients become surprised upon discovering that an estimated one out of every two Americans will suffer from arthritis during their lives. The debilitating and often painful condition can hit anyone, ranging from the very young to mature individuals. Some patients experience only mild discomfort while others suffer sever pain, sometimes resulting in deformed joints, decreased mobility, bodily weakness, depression and fatigue. Common specific symptoms can include a decrease in joint mobility, swelling, or similar symptoms as a result of climate change. The initial symptoms may occur in the distal fingers and the base of the thumbs.

Arthritis Causes

Genetics: Some patients experience what doctors call a "predisposition" to degenerative joint disease due to genetic factors passed from their parents or ancestors. Researchers list this as the most common arthritis, called "osteoarthritis," with symptoms usually emerging during a patient's mature years.

Hormone Imbalance: A variety of factors including stress, adrenal imbalance or excess caffeine can lead to hormonal imbalances—which, in turn, can generate various forms of arthritis.

Immunity: Weakened immune systems can lead the body vulnerable to the onset of certain forms of arthritis. Underlying factors here include certain types of bacteria that can generate the condition. Rarer specific types include rheumatoid, psoriatic and septic arthritis.

Lifestyle: The overuse of specific joints or injuries from a variety of causes such as sporting injuries, repetitive motion generates long-term stress that can lead to arthritis.

Swelling: Inflammation hampers tendon and joint function, leading to arthritic symptoms.

Additional Considerations

Researchers in recent years say they've increasingly found a link between arthritis and stress, particularly stemming from emotional or mental imbalances. Some patients benefit from stress-reduction techniques. (See the Stress section)

Arthritis Treatments

Take plenty of healthful minerals and vitamins derived from nutritional foods. Vitamin C serves as one of the most formidable treatments, thanks largely to its ability to reduce inflammation while aiding the re-growth of cartilage. Ingest ample levels of magnesium and zinc, while also taking vitamins E and B6. Other helpful factors of treatments:

Enzymes: Particularly among patients also suffering from ulcers, after first checking with your doctor, take enzymes at levels higher than the usually recommended dose.

Natural: Generating results previously considered impossible, some patients benefit from shark or bovine cartilage with large amounts of substances that accelerate cartilage production in people, such as chondroitin glucosamine, MSM and SAM-E. Cartilage also re-grows from krill supplements.

Immunity: Take steps to boost your immune system, essential because arthritis stems from autoimmune disease. Effective foods or herbs for boosting immunity include spirulina, olive leaf extract and maca root.

Drink: Lots of lignite-activated water can help.

Key substances: Additional substances should include: glucosamine and chondroitin sulfates—added with S-adenosylmethionine—assisting in the body's absorption of glucosamine; high-potency fish oils; and green-lipped mussels. In addition, a form of dimethyl sulfoxide (DMSO)—methylsulfonylmethane—can treat with minimal side effects various kinds of arthritis, particularly the osteo and rheumatoid forms.

Asthma

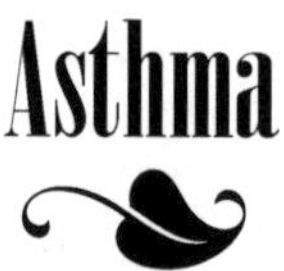

Bronchial Spasms

Also see the Allergies and Bronchitis sections

Asthma hails as the most common medical condition suffered by children under age 17. One of the top ten generators of hospitalization and disease among adults also stems from asthma. Besides the buildup of mucus in the lungs, frequent symptoms range from chest tightness and wheezing to difficulty breathing.

Asthma related suffocation kills an estimated 5,000 Americans yearly. The two most common forms of asthma include the "acute" variety, which hits suddenly—often with little or no warning. By contrast, acute asthma usually lasts for only brief periods of just a few hours—usually less severe than chronic asthma yet with continual symptoms, often lasting weeks to months.

Asthma Causes

Doctors often blame asthma on airborne allergens that enter the body through the mouth rather than the nose. Secondarily, the body's hypersensitivity to particular allergens or inadequate immunity sometimes accelerates, increasing the probability that the allergens will adversely impact the lungs. The specific causes that ignite these conditions can include cold air, food allergies, stress, exertion, poor nutrition, and drugs.

Additional Considerations

Concentrated breathing techniques have helped many asthma patients. This method strives to make breathing easier by using mind power to regulate breathing. Many people have benefited from a white powder containing yamoa from Africa, with positive results sometimes starting about ten days after a daily intake regimen begins.

Asthma Treatments

Supplements: Take what homeopaths call "oxygenating supplements," which accelerate or trigger the amount of oxygen entering the bloodstream. Containing more oxygen than any other plant, gel derived from aloe vera of the non-rind variety can produce a great drink. Other vitamins and minerals helpful in opening blood vessels and aiding circulation include ginkgo biloba oil, beta-carotene, B vitamins, Vitamin A and 50 milligrams three times daily of dimethyl-glycine. Carbon-activated water can help.

Bodily support: Strengthen immunity with nutrient-rich food, spirulina, Echinacea, and olive leaf extract. To boost the adrenal glands, take pantothenic acid with 150 milligrams of adrenal tissue twice daily.

Irritants and relief: Avoid irritating foods such as wheat products and dairy, both known to exacerbate allergies including asthma. Meantime, open bronchial passageways with various herbs and essential oils. These include: chamomile essential oils for relaxing bronchial spasms; bronchodilators such as pine essential oils, spearmint and peppermint; skullcap herbs; and herbal teas containing theophylline-like compounds.

Astigmatism

Also see sections on Cataracts, Macular Degeneration

People with astigmatism suffer poor or blurred vision. This occurs when the eye becomes oval shaped rather than round. Healthy eyes are round. By contrast, the oval shape of astigmatism forces the eye to focus on numerous points rather than one.

Besides blurred vision, the most common symptoms are eye pain, headaches and fatigue. Worsening matters, many people with astigmatism complain of fuzzy or blurry lines, gradually hampering depth perception. Straight lines sometimes appear distorted or even crooked.

Astigmatism Causes

Scientists admit they have been unable to identify a universal exact cause. The eye's cornea gradually loses its natural roundness. Some researchers believe that poor posture and frequently tilting the head can cause perception problems and astigmatism.

Additional Considerations

Some health experts insist that significant benefits in overall eye health can occur when patients exercise their eyes throughout the day—resting the eyes at least five minutes in every half-hour period, boosting overall energy while relaxing your gaze. Among other frequent eye exercises: regularly blinking to reduce strain, rolling the eyes in full circular motions down and up—in five minute daily sessions; in 20-minute to 30-minute sessions, rapidly refocusing from near to far; and regular meditative or rest sessions.

Astigmatism Treatments

The various treatment options each have varying degrees of risk. Invasive surgical procedures developed and improved in recent years include photo reactive keratomy or PRK, and Lasik surgery. Among potential negative side effects are impaired vision acuity, dry eyes, sensations of halos that surround lights, chronic dry eye, subjecting the body to potential free radical damage, and retina tears that can damage the optic nerve.

Rather than risk surgical complications, some patients choose natural cures and remedies. Embracing the "ayurvedic theory," numerous health professionals believe that digestive imbalances cause vision problems. Natural remedies here range from antioxidant vegetables, plus Ayurvedic herbs including licorice, trimhala and amla—while also regularly exercising the eyes.

Homeopaths believe that specific vitamins and supplements can significantly lessen such vision problems. Besides Vitamin A, Vitamin E and B complex vitamins, some homeopaths prescribe selenium, zinc, zeaxthanin, beta-carotene, flavonoids, taurine, selenium, riboflavin and N-acetyl-cystine or NAC.

Overall eye health often improves significantly when enjoying a healthy, balanced diet. Food selections often deemed helpful include organic egg yolks, leafy green vegetables, and many antioxidants like red grapes, citrus fruits, Goji berries, Acai berries, and unsweetened cocoa loaded with natural flavonoids and antioxidants.

Some health professionals recommend re-educating or exercising the eye, starting with relaxing the body and mind amid frequent breaks from regular activities. Tactics include meditating or walking, occasionally closing the eye while concentrating on "receptive awareness" and focusing on detailed scenery with eyes open.

Athletes Foot

Also see sections on Nail Fungus and Infections (Bacteria)

Commonly called "athletes foot," this foot fungus often strikes people who frequently exercise or engage in sports, running or exercise. Millions of people frequently suffer from this common condition. Fungal growth affects the foot's skin and sometimes toenails. Patients can suffer from cracking, scaling, stinging, burning and itching. The skin between the soles of the feet and toes commonly becomes inflamed.

Athlete's Foot Causes

Within the gastrointestinal tract a systemic yeast overgrowth or "candidiasis" can occur, resulting in natural imbalances throughout the body—possibly leading to fungal infections. Fixing this imbalance sometimes eliminates athlete's foot. Other common culprits leading to athlete's foot include exposure in locker rooms and swimming pools, or improper foot hygiene.

Additional Considerations

Some practitioners of natural health remedies report that fungus growth often reduces among patients who eat diets low in dairy products while rich in whole grains and raw foods. Also avoid yeast-producing foods or beverages like beer, wine, cheese, bread and pickled foods. Dietary supplements that often prove helpful include vitamins A, C and E and B-complex, zinc, acidophilus and bifidobacteria.

Athlete's Foot Treatments

Some health experts recommend applying natural or synthetic oils to infected areas. Oils derived from geranium, tea trees and patchouli are often deemed helpful. Flower essences such as crab apple can help. Among herbal extracts and combinations are grapefruit seed extract topically applied; diluted tea tree oil with lavender oil, or calendula; pau d'arco from wet tea bags that have been soaked ten minutes; honey mixed with garlic before being topically applied; and antifungal oregano, garlic, myrrh or pine oils.

Autoimmune Disorder

Also see Immune System Health

Within healthy people the body's immune system naturally has the ability to protect bodily tissues by fighting foreign invaders. Yet in some individuals the body's immune system fails to discern or identify differences between the body's own cells and those of invaders. Such difficulties cause the immune system to attack the body's tissues, the condition called "autoimmune disorder."

A wide variety of diseases and adverse health conditions involve autoimmune disorder. Some of the most common include Crohn's disease, sprue, chronic thyroiditis, scleroderma, Addison's disease, pernicious anemia, rheumatoid arthritis, lupus, vitiligo, Sjogrens syndrome, Lou Gehrig's disease, and multiple sclerosis. Some researchers also think Type 1 Diabetes is an autoimmune disorder.

Catastrophic or debilitating health conditions can result from autoimmune disorders as the immune system attacks the body's vital organs or tissues, and cells. Essential bodily areas sometimes hurt include the muscles, pancreas, endocrine glands and thyroid. Specific symptoms and long-term prognosis vary depending on severity.

Autoimmune Disorder Causes

Overall, scientists admit they have been unable to determine why the immune system attacks the body. Some researchers believe these patients often suffer a subtle change in cells that wreck the body's cells from recognizing parts of "itself," or from a "genetic predisposition" or an inherited biological propensity to suffer from such conditions.

Autoimmune Disorder Treatments

Increase: Increase consumption of foods high in omega-3 fatty acids such as cold-water fish like wild salmon or chia seeds, tofu, walnuts, and flaxseed oil.

Avoid: Remove gluten from the diet, avoid wheat based cereals and breads, replacing them with quinoa or rice-based cereals, breads and gluten-free pasta.

Assist: Help boost the body's natural immunity with folic acid supplements and Vitamin B12, improving vitiligo. Vitamins C and D have helped autoimmune disorders, curtailing over-activity of the immune system.

B

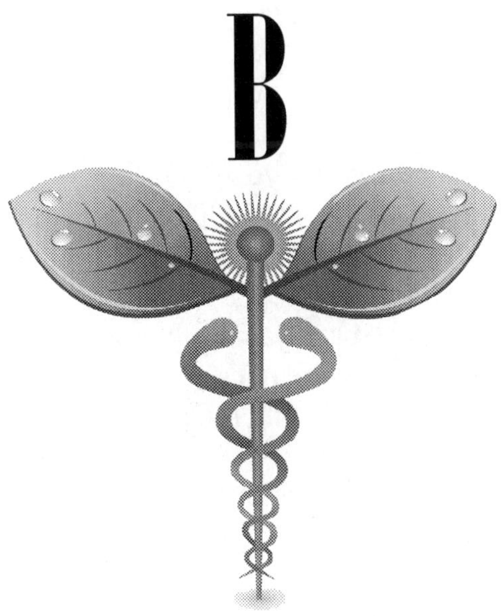

Back Pain

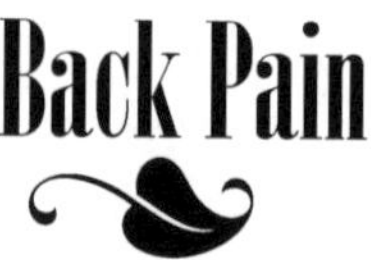

Also see Muscle Cramps, Arthritis, Liver and Gallbladder Health

Back pain has been listed as the second most common reason why U.S. citizens visit a doctor. Medical professionals estimate that at least four out of every five people will suffer back pain during their lifetimes. Some patients get highly addictive or dangerous pain medications that fail to address the primary underlying causes of back pain. Many patients get steroid injections, epidural shots, surgeries or other invasive procedures, often repeating this process for years.

However, numerous medical industry observers complain that many back surgeries are unnecessary, with adverse symptoms often reappearing within four years. Homeopathic remedies strive to naturally "cure" back pain rather than mask symptoms. Chiropractic adjustments sometimes eliminate pain and acupuncture may also give lasting relief.

Back pain sometimes worsens over time, leading some homeopaths to recommend "healthy lifestyle" strategies for preventing back pain and for maintaining good health.

Back Pain Causes

Besides poor posture, common causes can include: insufficient exercise or physical activity; excessive body weight; sleeping in unhealthful positions; muscle strains caused by exercise and work; inflammation of tendons, fascia or joints. These conditions are sometimes caused by medications, injury or the deterioration of bodily areas around ligaments; misaligned hips, shoulders or spine; liver toxicity or liver disease (sometimes caused by alcohol); and spinal problems such as scoliosis.

Additional Considerations

Some homeopaths or other practitioners of natural remedies rub natural substances such as cramp bark, lobelia on affected areas to reduce pain. Helpful herbs taken orally include cat's claw, yucca root, wild yam, rosemary and feverfew—but only in instances that do not involve kidney toxicity. Use detoxifying treatments and saunas in those instances. Other potential remedies to be used only under professional supervision include acupuncture, bodywork such as massages, chiropractic, the Feldenkrais Method for correcting posture, hydrotherapy, oxygen therapy, Ayurveda, Traditional Chinese Medicine and far infrared mats and saunas.

Back Pain Treatments

The most effective treatments involve "preventing the problem" with frequent stretching, exercise and healthy eating. So, pay close attention to posture and movement. Sleep in spacious, comfortable conditions. At work or in your vehicle, sit only in seats that provide good back support. This is particularly essential for overweight people. Also, avoid alcohol or prescription medicines that can build liver toxicity, leading to back pain.

Also, identify the type of pain that you suffer before using remedies. Muscular imbalance causes pointed sharp lower back pain—often easily cured by slow and long stretching exercise, usually on a floor. Stretching or movement that intensifies or exacerbates pain indicates spinal or tissue damage that requires anti-inflammatory remedies.

Kidney problems sometimes cause aching in the mid- or lower back, generating a need to have these organs and the liver cleaned. Helpful and powerful remedies here can include green tea, Devil's Claw, and milk thistle.

Use effective natural anti-inflammatory vitamins, supplements and foods. These include garlic, and cinnamon and supplements of fish oil and turmeric. Supplements that help prevent back pain contain calcium, magnesium, glucosamine, coenzyme Q10, SAM-e and vitamins A and C.

To stimulate the body's natural collagen production, thereby growing connective tissue including ligaments, some back pain sufferers use "prolotherapy"—the injection of an "irritant solution" in the painful area. Specifically, this can eliminate some back pain problems that had resulted from damaged ligaments. Within the body the injection ignites an inflammatory response, creating a "domino effect" in which the body rebuilds connective tissue.

Bad Breath

Halitosis

Also see the GERD section

At some point in life certain foods cause almost every person to experience bad breath in the morning or throughout the day. Labeled by doctors as "halitosis" or "oral malodor," this problem motivates Americans to collectively spend millions of dollars yearly on remedies in efforts to avoid offending relatives, colleagues or friends. The most commonly used remedies have little effect on the underlying cause, everything from drops and strips to mouth wash, chewing gum and mints. Regular flossing is a must.

Bad Breath Causes

Food or bacteria in the mouth cause this problem, signaling the need for effective oral hygiene. Although brushing and cleaning the mouth usually helps, a lack of eating healthful foods can generate stomach acids that trigger bad breath. Insufficient amounts of normal fluids in the mouth can cause similar odor as dryness creates conditions for bacteria to grow and spread. Prescription drugs and dehydration are common culprits. Such conditions also can threaten dental health. Poor oral hygiene habits contribute.

Bad Breath Treatments

For cases of chronic bad breath, improve the diet, focusing on healthy foods while avoiding junk food, before cleaning in chronological order the colon, intestines, liver and kidneys. Drink ample quantities of pure water for all types of bad breath, hydrating the mouth and body—removing foul-smelling bacteria from the tongue. Brush baking soda and hydrogen peroxide on your tongue using a toothbrush, particularly where bacteria and food particles accumulate way back near the throat. Especially when dry mouth causes chronic bad breath, stimulate natural saliva production either by avoiding drugs that cause the problem or using toothpaste, rinses or gum.

Bee Stings and Insect Bites

Bee Sting Hypersensitivity

Most people experience only temporary discomfort when stung by bees. Normal reactions caused by bee sting venom include redness, swelling and itching that usually lasts only a few hours. Avoid panicking if bees or wasps land on or buzz around you. Most of the time these creatures fly away without attacking, upon discovering you lack what they crave such as pollen and bright colors. Perfumes, hairsprays and foods may attract them.

Bee Sting Symptoms

Scientists have estimated that about one person out of every 1,000 has a dangerous hypersensitivity to bee sting venom. Such conditions impose a risk that bee stings will trigger extreme allergic reactions or even death. The most serious reactions that generate immediate medical help include impaired vision, breathing problems, nausea and swelling of the tongue.

Some of the worst symptoms begin occurring within hours

after a sting or multiple stings, including lymph gland swelling, fever and joint pain. Unless they are extremely venomous, the bites of other insects can cause similar symptoms, plus diarrhea, neck swelling, dizziness, fainting and swelling. Seek medical help when these occur.

Bee Sting and Insect Bite Treatments

Take an antihistamine to relieve pain, never grabbing any extended part of the stinger. Instead, flick the stinger out using a credit card, knife or other object that has an edge. Put ammonia or ice on the wound. Cold remedies slow the spread of poisons while providing relief. Cover the wound with a alkali paste comprised of crushed aspirin mixed with a small amount of water, meat tenderizer, toothpaste, bentonite clay, and baking soda.

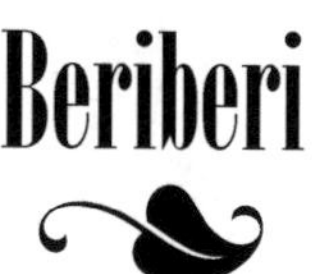

Wernicke-Korsakoff Syndrome

The B-vitamin deficiency commonly called “beriberi” can gradually lead to cardiovascular, physical and mental problems. The many symptoms can include whiteheads on the upper face or torso, difficulty warding off the common cold, memory loss, fatigue, irritability, vomiting, mental confusion, and a rapid heart rate. Heart attacks can occur in extreme cases. A significant reduction in blood flow to the head occurs in cardiovascular beriberi, “Wernicke-Korsakoff Syndrome.”

Beriberi Causes

The primary cause is failing to eat adequate amounts of Vitamin B1, called “thiamine,” or an inability to effectively ingest this substance caused by liver disease, gastrointestinal problems, severe stress, food allergies or parasites. Beriberi also can occur when the body loses or fails to use Vitamin B1. Besides stress and genetic predisposition, common causes involve the body expelling or failing to adequately use B1 or an overactive thyroid or "hyperthyroidism," severe fevers, breastfeeding, food allergies such as wheat intolerance, parasites, or intestinal damage caused by toxins including drugs or alcohol.

Beriberi Treatments

Eat foods rich in B vitamins such as yogurt, nuts, seeds, leafy green vegetables, brown rice, raw fruits and whole grains. Drinking excessive amounts of water at mealtime can flush out vital thiamin. Alleviate symptoms with Vitamin C, flower essences, and sulfur. Nutrient-dense "super food" containing bee pollen, maca, spirulina and other healthful substances can lessen or eliminate symptoms.

Bird Flu

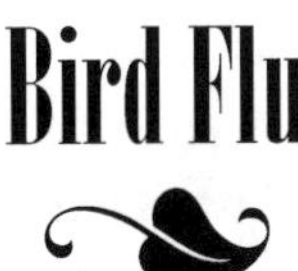

Avian Blu / Avian Influenza

Also see Infection (Viral)

Scientists estimate that 1 million people die yearly worldwide from the flu, including 36,000 Americans. History's worst simultaneous worldwide flu epidemic killed an estimated 50 million people worldwide, including 675,000 Americans. Many experts predict that it's just a matter of time before another pandemic strikes. Yet some researchers insist there is no way to predict if such an event will occur.

Several organizations including the World Health Organization and the National Centers for Disease Control closely monitor the development and potential spread of bird flu. Researchers worry that bird flu will develop into a human-to-human variety, spreading rapid-fire worldwide before entire societies and individuals take adequate precautions.

Bird Flu Transmission

Contaminated feces, nasal secretions and saliva are often considered the primary contributing factors in spreading bird flu. This apparently happens via direct contact with these substances, or when a bird touches or gets close to contaminated surfaces. Many researchers think that migratory birds could spread the virus worldwide. Previous epidemics began in regions of the Far East or Southeast Asia where people and animals live in close proximity. Such conditions apparently increase the likelihood that the virus will mutate from animals to humans.

Research indicates that infections suffered by humans result from people coming into contact with birds. Some doctors also fear that other animals, particularly cats, might also spread bird flu to people. This generates added concern because cats have frequent contact with birds and humans.

Additional Considerations

As with most infectious diseases and viruses, thorough hand washing can stop or curtail the spread of flu. Avoid foods, substances or behavior that weakens or lowers the immune system. These include alcohol, smoking, caffeine, drugs and dairy products. Antibiotics will fail to eliminate bird flu because such influenza is caused by a virus rather than bacteria.

Preventative Treatments

The best way to avoid getting the flu is to eat antiviral nutrients while also increasing blood alkalinity. This creates an environment hostile to the virus. Among nutrients that can help are olive leaf extract, Indian Echinacea, skullcap herbs, raw garlic, the natural adaptogen Siberian ginseng, oregano oil, Citricidal grapefruit extract, lysine, Vitamin C, colloidal silver, zinc, and immune-boosting, nutrient-rich foods such as purple or dark red berries and dark green leafy vegetables. These include wheat grass, rhygrass and algae.

Blood Pressure

(High) Hypertension

Also see Cholesterol, Weight (Over), Cardiovascular Health

Blood pressure measures the systolic and diastolic pressure between pulses. Scientists say there is no universal "ideal" blood pressure level for the entire population. Among individuals the concept of "normal" in this regard may vary. Ranges from 90/60 to 139/89 are considered normal for most individuals. People should take careful preventative measures and regularly monitor this condition if their blood pressure is in the high range.

Shortness of breath after mild exertion is one of the few symptoms of hypertension. Doctors consider hypertension as a signal of health issues including bad eating habits, excess weight and nervous stress. Particularly when left untreated, hypertension can lead to heart problems, brain damage and kidney failure—while increasing chances for blindness, stroke and heart attack.

High Blood Pressure Causes

Instances of high blood pressure increase with advanced age, particularly after age 60 when arteries start stiffening. This generally causes the lower of the two measurement numbers to increase, but not everyone in this age range experience such symptoms. Besides stress, smoking and caffeine, other contributors likely to exacerbate high blood pressure include excessive weight that forces the heart to work too much. Additional dangers emerge from trans fat or saturated fats and sugary or starchy foods. All these causes force the heart to beat harder and faster in order to supply the blood with adequate oxygen. Diabetes mellitus and chronic renal disease are important precursors.

Additional Considerations

Inadequate amounts of calcium, potassium, magnesium, and Vitamin C can raise blood pressure. So be sure to take healthful amounts of them on a regular basis.

Blood Pressure Treatments

Most involving lifestyle and diet, many strategies can effectively reduce high blood pressure. Some of the fastest-acting natural remedies include eliminating caffeine and smoking, while lowering stress, decreasing sodium intake, losing weight, exercising more under professional guidance, decreasing sugar and starch intake, and eating food that helps regulate blood pressure. These include raw onions, garlic and pure cocoa of the dark or bittersweet chocolate varieties. Prune juice, pears, peaches and other potassium-rich foods including bananas help boost this effort. Studies also show dramatic reductions in high blood pressure thanks to sesame oil. Saunas and hot baths can generate sweating that eliminates toxins from the body. Studies indicate that yoga and medication are excellent ways to reduce blood pressure.

Blood Pressure

(Low) Hypotension
Also see Thyroid Imbalance
Adrenal Insuffiency

Less common and usually less potentially serious than high blood pressure, hypotension is sometimes "mistakenly" considered healthy by some people. Yet low blood pressure can cause numerous health problems including sensitivity to cold weather, fainting, dizziness when suddenly standing or sitting, low physical energy, circulation problems, and skin disorders.

Low Blood Pressure Causes

Many researchers list hypotension as hereditary, yet other factors include habitually or chronically taking low, shallow breaths, diet, hypothyroidism, "adrenal burnout" and dehydration.

Low Blood Pressure Treatments

Enjoy lots of vigorous exercise and take plenty of dark chocolate or cocoa, often significant in regulating high blood pressure and low blood pressure. Eat increased amounts of spices like cayenne, turmeric, and curry, while keeping any possible thyroid imbalance in check with selenium, walnuts and kelp.

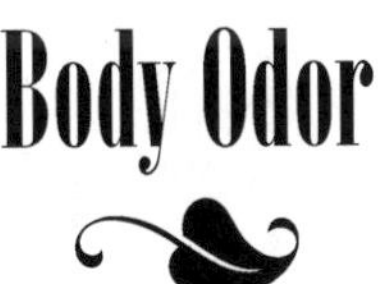

Bromhidrosis

Many people understandably become surprised upon discovering that antiperspirant products sold over-the-counter in drug stores contain harmful toxic metals. Yet many people feel dependent on such products, which usually emit pleasant aromas.

Rather than risk disease and a bodily degeneration caused by such toxins, people need to realize the underlying causes of offensive body odor—before regularly taking natural remedies to correct or prevent the problem. The offensive stench of body odor emanates from bacteria on hair and skin. The worst bodily areas are moist, covered by clothes—particularly the feet, groin and armpits.

Body Odor Causes

Sweat usually sparks the condition, except in instances where the person has toxic levels of heavy metals, drugs, alcohol or other microscopic materials. Sweat accelerates bacterial growth, particularly on the hair and the skin as well. The odor emanates from the bacteria rather than sweat, which serves as the breeding ground of these biological organisms at the anal area, underarms, groin, breasts, palms and even the forehead.

Some of the most offensive odors build up when thick and sticky underarm sweat becomes a yellowish breeding ground for bacteria. This problem intensifies when the bacteria interact with underarm hair follicles. Numerous factors combine to determine the severity and duration of the odor, including weather, diet and the individual's DNA. Some people emit more intense body odor than others.

Additional biological triggers or factors range from medications and smoking to alcohol and diet. People who eat lots of meat sometimes emit certain distinctive odors, stemming from their body's processing of animal fats. Garlic and garlic products produce the most consistent malodorous results. Aluminum toxicity may occur from overuse of deodorants and creams.

Additional Considerations

Contrary to popular belief among many people worried about body odor, sweat is actually a "good" rather than a "bad" thing. Perspiration serves the vital function of cooling the body. So, you have added reason to avoid toxic antiperspirants. Instead, use natural oils and deodorants to smell clean or fresh. Antiperspirants and deodorants have vastly different functions. Antiperspirants block or prevent natural detoxification and healthful sweating; deodorants generally emit pleasant smells rather than blocking sweat.

Body Odor Treatments

Drink healthful and continuous daily amounts of water to help cleanse the body and organs of toxins. Bathe regularly using natural, non-toxic soaps, and regularly change into clean clothes. Wash your hair, change into dry shoes and socks regularly as needed. Avoid alcohol and unnecessary drugs. Some adults should clean their bodies before going into public places after sex—particularly women who have intense or multiple orgasms.

Breast Cancer

Also see Weight (Over), Hormone Imbalance

Breast cancer remains one of the top 10 killers of women in the United States. The instance of breast cancer among women sometime during their lives is a whopping one out of eight. The instance of the disease has climbed markedly since 1960, when one percent of women suffered breast cancer. Despite significant overall medical advances in the past half century, the instance in breast cancer in women has grown to 12 percent.

Regular annual breast examinations serve as the best most reliable method of catching the disease early enough for treatments to be effective. Women from age 45 to 55 have the greatest risk, and thus a greater need for such tests, particularly individuals whose relatives had the disease. This is called the perimenopausal period.

Regular self-examination is a priority, along with annual mammograms by medical professionals. The most significant potential signals that women should watch for include sensitivity or pain in lymph nodes or lumps in the underarms, nipple discharges, bleeding, nipple pain, changes in nipple appearance, dimply skin around the breast, and breast swelling.

Breast Cancer Causes

Poor nutrition is a suspected trigger among some individuals. Many women are predisposed to getting breast cancer for genetic reasons. Yet four out of five females with breast cancer have no family history of the disease. Many researchers insist there is no evidence that that natural hormonal changes that women experience when aging cause the disease, although most females with breast cancer get the disease after age 50. Rather than hormonal changes, some researchers suspect early puberty, obesity, or having children in their 40s or late 30s. Higher risks also occur among women who take specific synthetic estrogens, drink or smoke, or do not breast feed.

Additional Considerations

Mammograms are increasingly controversial, some researchers claiming that such examinations actually increase the likelihood of getting breast cancer. Various studies have claimed that women who get annual mammograms have a 52 percent risk of dying from breast cancer. Yet many health professionals and organizations including the American Cancer Society advocate regular mammograms—which expose the body to radiation, a known carcinogen. To avoid such danger, some women choose to have their breasts examined via non-invasive thermograms that lack radiation.

Breast Cancer Treatments and Prevention

Many physicians cite the disturbing fact that the rates of all types of cancer have increased along with the rise in artificial foods and chemicals added to meals. Some medical professionals, particularly homeopaths, urge strategies to remove toxins from the body while boosting health with vitamin and mineral supplements.

This tactic involves avoiding milk loaded with artificial hormones, spending time outdoors without sunscreen to get plenty of natural Vitamin D, and loading up on B and E vitamins from foods and supplements. Eat nutrition-rich food to fortify overall immune system health, while avoid toxic antiperspirant products.

Just as important, women with breast cancer or who strive to prevent the disease should eat soy products loaded with natural phytoestrogens. Supplements deemed helpful in preventing cancer including that of the breast contain natural antioxidants. The most helpful include conjugated linoleic acid, spirulina, chlorella, selenium and adrenal extracts. Loaded with beta-glucans and enzymes, maitake mushroom extract fights cancer, bacteria, fungus and virus. To boost the body's T and NK cells that battle cancer, take green tea and Pycnogenol. Avoid all synthetic hormones.

Bronchitis

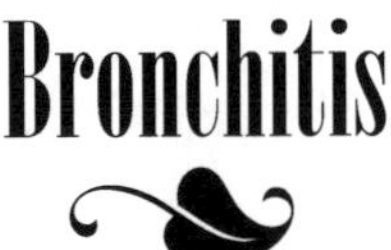

Also see Coughs, Asthma

Bronchitis can develop into a potentially serious condition leading to pneumonia. Only medical professionals can diagnose bronchitis, when inflammation of the bronchial airways is accompanied by a wet, dry or deep cough. The flu, viral infections, sinusitis or a cold sometimes generate acute bronchitis. Severe or long-lasting bronchitis sometimes generates breathlessness, wheezing, the excessive production of phlegm or mucus, fever and chills, and finally life-threatening pneumonia.

Bronchitis Causes

Numerous underlying factors are often blamed, such as environmental toxins, food allergies, bacteria and viral infections. Second-hand smoke and smoking sometimes contribute. The overall problem become dangerous, even when relatively mild or short durations of this condition trigger significant infections and pneumonia—particularly in instances where bronchitis goes untreated. Reflux disease is often a hidden cause.

Additional Considerations

To prevent or reverse recurring bronchitis, take healthful nutritional supplements that contains vitamins A and C, plus selenium, zinc and beta-carotene. Many homeopaths also recommend bromelain, thymus gland extract, colloidal silver, N-acetylcysteine, olive leaf and colostrum.

Bronchitis Treatments

Acupuncture, oxygen therapy, and detoxification therapy are among alternative therapies sometimes deemed helpful. A wide variety of effective remedies include moving to or creating a "clean-air" environment, changing diet, herbs, aromatherapy and checking for food allergies. Implement such positive changes or treatments before or during bronchitis episodes. Avoiding sugars, wheat, soft drinks, and corn can play a significant role while drinking lots of clean water. Enjoy ample portions of organic foods, while limiting dairy, eggs, caffeine, and bananas, which stimulate mucus production. Eat lots of organic whole foods, a vegan diet that eliminates dairy and meat.

Among a vast range of herbs helpful in treating bronchitis are peppermint, goldenseal, anise, astragalus, coldstood, garlic, diluted grapefruit seed extract, Saint John's wort, Echinacea and propolis that has been dropped into the throat area before inhaling the vapors. High-dose Vitamin C administered via IVs also may be beneficial.

Bruising

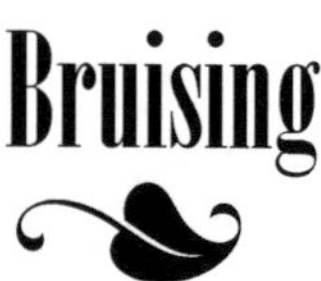

Contusions / Ecchymoses

Besides accidents and war wounds, lifestyle behaviors most typically associated with bruising are physical activities like sports and youthful roughhousing. Accidental injuries such as falls or bumping into things also causes bruising—blood capillary damage at or near the wound, blood amassing at or near the body surface in the afflicted area. Bruises commonly disappear three to 10 days after injury. Antioxidants and Vitamin C can help accelerate healing.

Additionally, bruising sometimes occurs without any apparent cause. Get a thorough physical examination when this happens. Some bruises, particularly when no injury has occurred, indicate a potential underlying problem—clotting disorders sometimes caused by low platelets, blood thinners or steroids. In addition, patients undergoing chemotherapy or suffering from leukemia or bone marrow cancer frequently have bruising. People older than 59 often have more bruising than younger people; many seniors have fragile blood vessels and thin skin.

Additional Considerations

Numerous homeopathic remedies lessen or remove bruising. When a dark wound heals slowly, apply sulfuric acid homeopathic. Ledum often helps, and arnica reduces discoloration or accelerates the disappearance of bruising.

Bruising Treatments

Besides applying apple cider or white vinegar on the bruise, eat foods rich in Vitamin C, antioxidants, and bioflavonoids. Also put lavender oil, camphor, hyssop or propolis tincture to the wound. For severe cases platelet transfusions or steroids may be necessary.

Burns

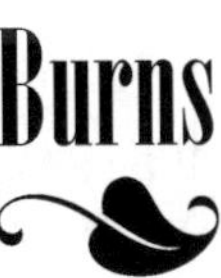

Blisters
Also see Sunburn

Direct exposure to fire, hot objects or heat from the sun causes the most burns. Touching stoves or ovens that are "on" can burn or dry the skin, generating scars, blisters, tissue damage and redness. Radiation, chemicals and electricity also cause burns.

The mildest burns, listed as "first-degree," only damage the skin's surface. These are red and usually heal naturally within several days after treatment with natural remedies. The more severe "second-degree" burns damage tissues beneath the skin, also harming nerves. Like "first-degree burns," such wounds of the second-degree usually can be treated at home—except in cases of children, who should be brought to medical facilities for care. The most severe burns are "third-degree," critically damaging or removing large sections of skin. Third-degree burns require immediate treatment from medical professionals, preferably at hospitals or critical care clinics. The quick application of treatments of third-degree burns also can sometimes help accelerate healing.

Additional Considerations

The starches of potato pulp, plantation pulp or extract can add moisture, cooling and soothing—cleaning, and also minimizing scars and blisters. Burns sometimes rob the body of minerals, which can be replaced by spirulina, bee pollen and mineral supplements. Use oregano oil drops to disinfect broken blisters. Creams containing silver are helpful.

Burn Treatments

Immediately use cold water to run over or soak the wound. Continue until pain diminishes. Cold water can prevent blisters, particularly when applied fast in sufficient quantities. Re-hydrate the dehydrated burn area with carbon-activated water or "Willard water." Put a few drops of Saint John's wort in water, which is then applied to the wound for cleaning. Cover the wound with papaya pulp or aloe vera pulp, preferably with a few drops of calendula or lavender oil to boost healing.

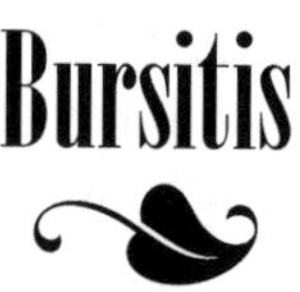

Also see Inflammation, Arthritis

This painful or achy condition erupts when cavities around tendons and muscles become inflamed. Synovial fluid fills these cavities, sometimes generating severe or prolonged inflammation that can generate long-term severe pain. Besides generating redness, swelling and localized muscle aches, bursitis can decrease motion in vital joints like the shoulders, hips and elbows—sometimes even rendering such regions immobile.

Bursitis Causes

The wide range of varied causes range from infection and gout to environmental toxins, calcium deposits that amass in the joints, trauma, physical injury, overuse of joints, allergies, osteoarthritis, deficiencies in Vitamin B12 or magnesium, and rheumatoid arthritis, inflammatory arthritis, post-traumatic arthritis, and sport injuries.

Additional Considerations

Some medical professionals strive to relieve bursitis patients' pain by injecting Vitamin B12. Supplements taken between meals to fortify or accelerate healing can contain Vitamin C, calcium, magnesium, proteolytic enzymes and bioflavonoid. Some patients report reduced or relieved symptoms thanks to alternative therapies like traditional Chinese medicine, acupuncture, bodywork, chiropractic, infrared mats and saunas.

Bursitis Treatments

Changing diet, topical applications, aromatherapy and hydrotherapy sometimes work. Such natural remedies often include drinking apple cider vinegar or filtered water, or ingesting honey preferably at bedtime. Eat food high in magnesium like yellow vegetables or dark leafy greens. Bursitis sufferers sometimes can benefit from juice supplements that contain equal portions of beet, carrot, cucumber and celery. To fortify digestion, have one tablespoon of cod liver oil within one or two hours before eating. Avoid "nightshade" vegetables like eggplant, tomatoes and potatoes.

Taken as tea or tinctures flower essence can be applied at least four times daily to painful areas. Ingredients recommended by homeopaths include aloe vera, horsetail, meadowsweet and willow bark. Rub cramp bark or lobelia on the affected area, and relieve pain and relax drinking chamomile tea. Additional helpful homeopathic treatments sometimes include Ruta grav, Arnica, Belladonna and Silicea.

Butter or Margarine

Hydrogenated Vegetable Oil / Trans Fat

Medical professionals, scientists and doctors continue to disagree on the possible negative impacts of margarine. Yet a steadily increasing number of studies identify negative health problems triggered by margarine. The danger is so severe that many homeopaths list margarine as extremely dangerous to health. Although butter and margarine have equal caloric levels, butter has higher fat levels per tablespoon—eight grams of saturated fats compared to five grams for margarine.

At least one study indicates that women who eat margarine have a 53-percent higher instance of heart disease than women who eat butter. In fact, although butter has more fat, it actually increases the body's ability to absorb nutrients from other foods. Margarine has only a few nutrition benefits, but only because those nutrients are added by machines. By contrast, experts say butter has numerous nutritional benefits.

The many negative impacts of margarine include: decreasing breast milk quality; lowering the body's immune responses; increasingly unhealthy cholesterol; boosting the probability of diabetes by decreasing insulin responses; and subjecting people to the type of fatty acids and trans fats that kill 30,000 Americans yearly.

Among other disturbing facts:

Synthetic: Change just one molecule in margarine and the result is plastic.

Dyes: Harmful toxic dyes are used to add yellow to margarine, which is initially black. The toxicity from these dyes can cause allergic reactions in almost everyone, including hyperactivity and attention deficit among children.

Arteries: Margarine forces a slick sludge to accumulate on arterial walls, blocking arteries—thereby leading to heart disease or potential death.

Danger warning: Even flies are "biologically smart" enough to avoid tubs of margarine that have been left in garages or shaded areas. Just as disturbingly, margarine never rots because the substance lacks nutrition. Nothing will grow on or in margarine, even microorganisms.

C

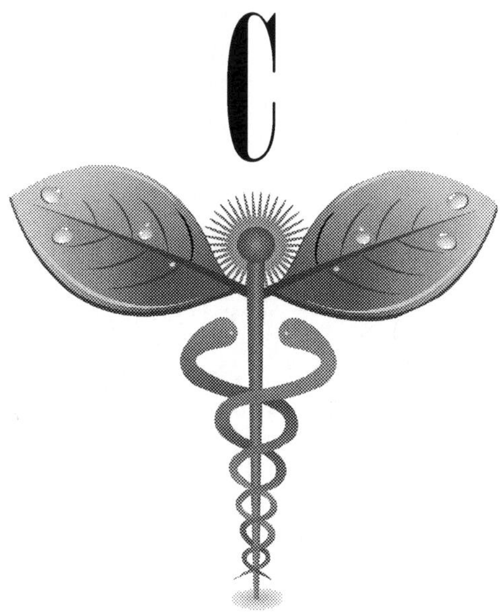

Cancer

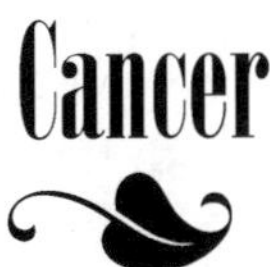

Also see Prostate Health, Breast Cancer

A mere half century ago most Americans considered any diagnosis of cancer as an automatic "death sentence." Of course many people today understand such a declaration is absurd.

Unlike in the mid-1900s, society today seems aware of the indisputable fact that a vast majority of cancer patients never die from the disease. Many of us in the 21st Century also know that huge medical advances have been made in the past 60 years.

However, although our current culture is far more knowledgeable about cancer, most everyday people lack any inkling of the biology involved in this disease—and even basics regarding the most likely causes.

Many people admit surprise upon learning researchers believe that most cancers do not erupt due to "inherited traits from the person's ancestors." To the contrary, most instances of this disease are caused by environmental toxins, plus dietary and lifestyle choices.

Cancer rates are relatively moderate or low in underdeveloped countries. By contrast, the percentages of people with the disease are far higher in developed countries that generate carcinogenic artificial substances and food preservatives.

At least some positive news is clear, though. Many types of the disease can be cured, often by using natural remedies. Consumers also can take measures to avoid known carcinogens.

Cancer Causes

Technically cancer is a mutation, the biological result of when something within the body's cells "goes wrong." Instead of growing and spreading as healthy cells, the mutations—called "cancer"—attack healthy body tissue as the disease spreads.

Scientists blame the formation of the damaged cell mutations on everything from carcinogenic substances that include smoking, asbestos, chemicals added to food, radiation, viruses and bacteria.

A person's lifestyle habits also can increase the likelihood of cancer. Alcohol can generate cancers of the stomach, breast, mouth, prostate and esophagus. A sedentary lifestyle and/or obesity clear a pathway for the formation of cancers in the colon, breast bladder and prostate. Tobacco triggers cancers in the upper body, particularly the lungs, mouth, sinuses.

Eating unhealthy foods that lack nutrition ravages the body's immunity, clearing a pathway for various types of cancer. Parasites, hepatitis and immune deficiencies are associated with numerous forms of cancer. Just as disturbing, a wide variety of manufactured and natural substances subject the human body to carcinogens.

Cancer Treatments

A vast array of natural remedies and lifestyle choices are available to prevent or to control cancer. The best ways to prevent this dreaded disease are to avoid carcinogenic chemicals, food additives, tobacco, alcohol, artificial sweeteners, radiation and bacteria.

Overweight people should steer clear of processed foods, meat, starches, sugar and saturated fat. While continually maintaining these vows, heavy people should eat more natural enzymes, proteins and amino acids.

With similar fervor, everyone should eat natural unprocessed foods proven to fight or prevent cancer. Besides garlic, broccoli and onions, the many powerful anti-cancer foods include carrots, cauliflower, cabbage, broccoli, tomatoes, romaine lettuce, spinach, kale—most high in lutein, a powerful antioxidant. (For more specific detail on healthy foods, get my popular selling book the "Forsythe Anti-Cancer Diet, available via all standard brick-and-mortar bookstores across North American and Europe, and from major online book and ebook retailers.)

Additional Considerations

Even while you're cancer-free, or if your body now contains the disease, take plenty of vitamins E and C, plus beta-carotene to fortify immunity. Purple and red berries provide ample essential antioxidants.

A variety of additional herbs and plants are sometimes recommended by practitioners of natural medicine—taken alone or in conjunction with chemotherapy to increase the probability of remission. Among the powerful natural substances that I often recommend are; vitamins B1, B2 and B12 contained in Poly-MVA along with amino acids, trace minerals and alpha-lipoic acid; and herbs derived from cats claw, pau d'arco, and paw-paw, and extracts from mistletoe or from the maitake, shiitake and reishi mushrooms.

Various "super-foods" help fight or prevent cancer. Alga Spirulina and alga chorella boost immunity, fortifying the body's natural killer cells that effectively fight cancer. Just as promising according to researchers an adrenal hormone—dehydroepiandrosterone (DHEA)—battles cancer of the lung, prostate, breast and colon when ingested, also preventing skin cancer when applied as a cream.

Additional Factors

Within the body cancer flourishes in an acidic environment, while most forms of the disease fail to live or thrive in highly alkaline conditions. Cancer usually fails to propagate in a systemic pH above 7 and especially greater than 7.5—but not always. Ideally, your blood should be balanced, toward alkaline, preferably in the 8-9 range. Foods most commonly blamed by homeopaths for creating overly acidic environments include fatty meats, sugars and highly processed carbohydrates.

Instead, eat lots of lean proteins in the mornings along with ample water. Green powders containing blue-green algae, barley, rye and wheat grass help push up alkalinity. Professional colon therapists can use coffee enemas to rid the body of carcinogens.

People everywhere also can reduce cancer risk factors by implementing stress- and anxiety-reduction methods described under Stress in this book.

Candida

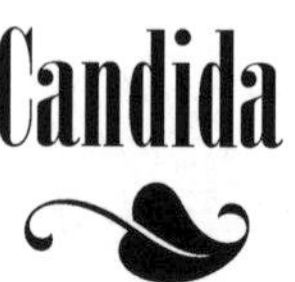

Candida Albicans / Thrush / Yeast Infection

Also see Infection (Bacteria), Colon and Intestinal Health

Three of every four women suffer from candida during their lifetimes, many experiencing this condition numerous times. Commonly called a "yeast infection," this involves a natural fungus within the bodies of almost every person. The fungus usually interacts normally with the body's flora without causing health problems. Yet sometimes the fungus grows too fast, creating the infections. Vaginal symptoms can include irritation, itching, and a thick, sour-smelling and milky vaginal discharge. Candida also sometimes causes rashes on the arms, or at various moisture-covered bodily areas such as the genitals, groin, buttocks, underarms and breasts. People of both genders can suffer from "thrush," when candida forms in the mouth, a painless but sometimes itchy or irritating condition that creates white patches on the tongue, cheeks and lips.

Candida Causes

The body's level of Candida go off balance when a person lacks sufficient levels of flora needed to counterbalance or keep that fungus "in check." The most common causes of candida beside poor diet and elevated blood sugars include antibiotics, chemotherapy, birth control pills, and AIDS medications. People suffering from diabetes, AIDS, CFIDs (chronic fatigue immune dysfunction) and fibromyalgia experience thrush more frequently than other individuals. In patients suffering from continual bouts of Candida, doctors consider the condition as a possible sign of immune deficiency syndromes, chronic fatigue or diabetes.

Additional Considerations

A controversial natural remedy has been used since the 1940s. The U.S. Food and Drug Administration has been trying to curtail or ban the use of oral colloidal silver—deemed by many homeopaths as a potentially powerful natural weapon that effectively treats candida. Contrary to the federal government's position on this issue, practitioners of natural medicine consider colloidal silver harmless when administered at safe, non-toxic levels during limited optimal time periods.

Candida Treatments

Standard allopathic physicians and particularly homeopaths usually employ two primary strategies. First, they remove yeast from the person's diet or environment. Second, the medical professionals introduce healthy flora into the person's diet. The diet restriction removes fermented foods from the diet, particularly cheese, soy sauce, wine and pickled dietary products. Patients also are urged to stop eating foods that cause blood sugar levels to increase, such as simple carbohydrates and sugar—substances that enable the candida yeast to thrive.

Foods that increase the body's healthful flora include yogurts that contain live dahi, kefir and cultures. Homeopaths recommend eating a variety of these cultures, plus probiotic cultures at least three times daily—consistently for at least one month. To remove candida rashes from various areas of the body apply oregano oil or garlic oil directly on the affected area at least three times daily. For best results, dilute these oils by at least one quarter by mixing in sweet almond oil or mineral oil. The application of these oils might initially create stinging sensations, a signal that the oils' antifungal properties are working as intended.

Cardiovascular Health

Arterial Stenosis / Atherosclerosis
Also see Weight (Over), Heart Disease, Cholesterol, Blood Pressure

The number one cause of death in Europe and the United States occurs when individually or in combination, adverse lifestyle or diet habits or hereditary generates the buildup of harmful cholesterol, plaque and fatty acids that endanger the heart and blood vessels. The excessive buildup of these substances can generate "atherosclerosis," restricting the vital and essential flow of blood to the brain and heart. Particularly when left unchecked over time the condition can lead to strokes, heart attacks or life-threatening heart conditions. Radical or invasive treatments often become required at the point when such negative conditions occur.

Rather than enable these adverse conditions to build within the body, people should strive to prevent cardiovascular and heart problems by eating healthy diets and making good lifestyle choices.

Cardiovascular Disease Causes

Besides harmful sugary, starchy diets high in saturated fats—the principal cause of such disease in the United States, people should strive to refrain from becoming overweight, a primary contributing factor. Such foods or body weight increases chances of high blood pressure, usually caused by stress, diet or disease; these factors, in turn, increases the chances of heart failure or other cardiovascular problems.

The aging process increases these dangers as arteries naturally stiffen, so strive to minimize this contributing factor by taking vitamins and antioxidants. Adverse triggering factors include a sedentary lifestyle, smoking and exposure to environmental toxins. Diabetes can boost sugar levels and cholesterol, leading to plaque buildup in arteries, elevated blood pressure and weight gain. Some people have a genetic or inherited predisposition to such problems, usually triggered by one or more of the known causes. Stress or hormonal imbalances also can make blood pressure high, contributing to cardiovascular disease.

Additional Considerations

Red wine decreases the potentially harmful stickiness of blood platelets while promoting a healthy heart. Loaded with beneficial bioflavonoid and antioxidants in moderation, red wine also inhibits the formation of "bad" cholesterol.

Cardiovascular Disease Treatments and Problem Prevention

Preventing cardiovascular problems or controlling such adverse conditions after they emerge hinge on a healthy diet. Everyone should avoid excess alcohol, curtail drug use, and stop smoking. Fortify the diet with heart-healthy omega-3 fatty acids found naturally in flaxseed oil and fish oils. Rather than coffee, enjoy green tea or green tea extract. Also, enjoy antioxidant rich foods including raw cocoa, garlic and soy.

To maintain healthy blood pressure and while promoting healthy cholesterol, eat lots of garlic. This lowers "bad" LDL cholesterol, while increasing "good" HDL cholesterol—while minimizing the possibility of deadly blood clots. Garlic naturally thins the blood. So, before taking garlic supplements, patients should consult with their health care professionals—particularly if taking blood-thinning drugs.

Health experts also urge patients to get exercise or engage in other stress-reducing activities like yoga, massage and saunas. Numerous natural supplements include: vitamins C, E, B3, B6 and B12; hawthorn berry extract; potassium; chromium; red yeast; magnesium; calcium; and L-carnitine, L-taurine, and L-arginine amino acids. Also helpful are curcumin, bioperine—a pepper extract—the pine bark extract pycnogenol, ribose, beta-carotene, and eicosapentaenoic acid.

Carpal Tunnel Syndrome

Cululative Trauma Disorder (CTC) / Repetitive Motion Syndrome / Tendonitis, also see Inflammation

Repetitive motion such a typing can lead to an adverse health condition called "carpal tunnel syndrome," particularly among women who are undergoing hormonal changes caused by menstruation, pregnancy or menopause. The hands suffer from extreme pain or restrict motion. The hands can feel as if they've "fallen asleep," while fingers and palms become numb. Some patients have difficulty making fists or gripping things, or feel burning and tingling sensations in the hands—which sometimes become highly sensitive to temperature.

CTS Causes

The median nerve within the carpal tunnel passageway between the wrist and hands becomes damaged, pinched or squeezed due to overuse, wreaking havoc on the vital nerves, controls the sensations of the middle fingers, palm and hand. Some people suffer CTS due to overuse of hands or the wrists, while other people who undergo similar repetitive motion never experience such problems. This leads some health professional to theorize that a combination of factors is involved, including hormone levels and whether the person has a naturally small carpal tunnel. A cancer of the plasma cells called "multiple myeloma" may cause this condition.

CTS Treatments

Stop or curtail repetitive movements if those were the primary cause. Take frequent breaks from stressful motions, change positions, and quickly massage the wrists. Eat natural anti-inflammatory foods such as vitamins E and C plus curry, turmeric and cayenne. Protect the nervous system by taking B vitamins.

Yoga exercises and acupuncture can help. Reduce inflammation in the carpal tunnel by eating curry, curcumin, cinnamon, aloe vera, yarrow root, skullcap and also a precursor to aspirin, white willow bark.

Cataracts

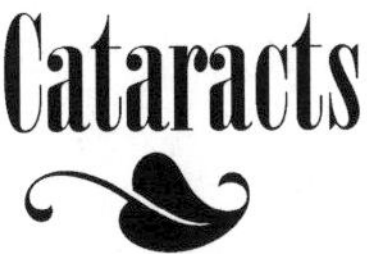

The blurry and sometimes opaque spots on the eye lens that curtail or hamper vision occur in most people older than age 70 and nearly half of people from 50-69. Modern surgical techniques often effectively repair or replace the lens. Homeopaths believe the best methods involve diet and lifestyle behaviors likely to prevent or minimize the severity of cataracts.

Cataract Causes

The aging process naturally leads to eye lens deterioration, while some people have a genetic predisposition to the condition. Sometimes the eyes get too much exposure to ultraviolet radiation from the sun or other sources. Another likely trigger involves hormonal imbalances caused by prescription drugs, diabetes and steroids.

Additional Considerations

Diets high in lutein reduce the risk of developing cataracts by about one-fifth in men and women, according to a Harvard Medical School Study. Natural foods with this nutrient include purple, yellow and red fruits, plus tomatoes, potatoes, romaine lettuce, dill, parsley, red peppers, kale, spinach, Swiss chard, mustard greens, collard, corn and carrots.

Cataract Treatments

Take antioxidants like pine bark extract called "Pycnogenol," and beta-carotene, and use carbon-activate water to wash the eyes every morning. Studies indicate that taking 500 milligrams of

Vitamin C daily continuously for at least a decade through age 59 helps lower by 57 percent the instance of cataracts at age 60 and older. Regularly drinking lots of water helps hydrate the eyes and the body.

Cellulite

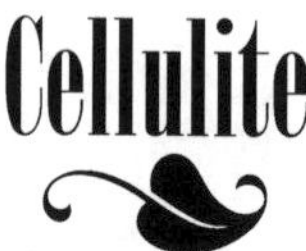

Also see Weight (Over), Liver and Gallbladder Health, Cardiovascular Health

That unsightly and strange-looking fat called "cellulite" afflicts a whopping 19 out of every 20 American women. Needless to say, this health issue has exploded into a national obsession, a persistent issue of health programs that strive to help females. Many women refuse to wear bathing suits, or seek help from the expensive and dangerous multi-billion-dollar surgical industry to remove the fat, a procedure called "liposuction."

Cellulite Causes

Many women who have cellulite are in the thin or moderate weight range, and most of course remain overweight. The bodies of women of all average weight levels form cellulite when the aging process or inadequate nutrition weakens blood vessels. This, in turn, decreases the effectiveness of blood to move nutrients. While the nutrients are transported toward the skin surface, fiber bands encapsulate the vessels before hardening. These bands build toward the skin, generating the unwanted, unsightly dimply cellulite.

Women experience this condition far more than men because the fat cells in females are more likely to bulge near the skin surface. Women "of color" experience cellulite less frequently than Caucasian females. Researchers also believe hormone levels also play a role. Even some men experience cellulite when estrogen levels increase. Cushing's Disease may cause this condition.

Compounding the problem, fat cells in both genders remain

even after fat is "burned off" within the cells. This factor gives formerly obese people the unwanted ability to easily regain weight. Health care professionals stress the need to burn energy before the body stores excess calories as fat. Besides reducing caloric intake or burning energy through exercise, there is no "cure" for cellulite. Even liposuction, a medical procedure that "sucks" fat from the body fails to permanently correct the condition. The mere removal of fat cells fails to prevent a recurrence of cellulite.

Cellulite Treatments

Always promote optimal cellular health by drinking lots of water. Regularly taking Vitamin C and bioflavonoid from seahawthorn, citrus fruit and mangoes reduces the possibility of cellulite by promoting healthy connective tissues. Also, eat fewer sugars, fats and carbohydrates, while increasing amino acids and proteins. Exercise daily to burn fat, particularly motions that accelerate breathing and sweating. For best results, eat before exercising rather than afterward. Eating before exercise triggers the body's catabolic process that burns fat, while eating afterward turns on the tissue-building anabolic system.

Chapped Lips

Angular Cheilitis

Almost everyone has experienced chapped lips, particularly when spending time outdoors relaxing, participating in sports or exercising. Exposure to the weather causes this condition, which ranges from extremely painful to mere annoyances.

Severe instances involve "angular cheilitis," painful lip cracks or splits—particularly at corners of the mouth—so painful that they bleed. Virus infections may cause this condition, rather than exposure to dry weather.

Chapped Lip Causes

Prone to chapping, sensitive epithelial tissue similar to what lines the anus covers the lips. Excessive moisture such as licking the lips, cold, allergenic lipstick and wind can cause chapping. The worst instances, angular cheilitis, occurs when excessively licking the lips, or from bacterial, or viral infections.

Chapped Lip Treatments

Petroleum-based products actually dry the lips, rather than moistening the tissue. The person's perceived need for continued use of these products generates ongoing revenue for the manufacturers. Natural substances work better, particularly gloss or lip balms made from vegetable or nut oils, beeswax or shea butter. Prevent chapping with B vitamins. Also benefit by applying ointments or oils loaded with vitamins E, D and A. Generous amounts can sometimes rapidly heal chapped lips. Used in conjunction with Vitamin E, antibacterial and antiseptic tea tree oil can effectively treat angular cheilitis.

Cholesterol

Bad Cholesterol (LDL) / Fat / Fatty Acids / Good Cholesterol (HDL) / Lipoproteins

Cholesterol comes in "good" and "bad" varieties. The situation becomes chemically complex in the liver, which processes both the good high-density HDL cholesterol and the bad LDL cholesterol. By eating lots of healthful nutrients people can help remove the bad LDL cholesterol from the body, preventing the substance from clogging the liver and arterial walls—thereby reducing the risk of coronary disease. The average person should strive to simplify the process, rather than getting fixated on scientific terms and substances ranging from saturated and unsaturated fats, VLDL cholesterol and triglycerides.

High Cholesterol Causes

The typical American diet that generates the greatest danger is critically high in salt, sugar, porocessed meat and fat. Food additives and exposure to toxins intensify the danger, along with stress and lifestyle choices like birth control pills, smoking, and caffeine. Foods loaded with starches and refined white sugar exacerbate the problem, causing inflammation while bad cholesterol sticks to arterial walls while oxidizing.

Additional Considerations

You should reduce soybean oil and walnut oil, although these are rich in beneficial LDL-reducing omega-3. These substances also feature omega-6, already contained in bulk in the typical unhealthful American diet.

High Cholesterol Treatments

Modify lifestyle choices while eating healthful foods and avoiding dangerous meals. High-fiber foods can help lower bad LDL cholesterol. Eating whole grains rather than refined grains is better for overall health, helping to prevent obesity and diabetes. Make the body use or burn off fats by taking potent Lipotropics like inositol, choline and methionine. Keep arterial walls clear by controlling bad LDL cholesterol, starting with a boost in soy, garlic and vegetables high in lutein. These include dill, red peppers, mustard greens, collard greens, carrots, corn, spinach, Swiss chard, kale, corn, tomatoes, potatoes, romaine lettuce, parsley, and blue or purple fruits. Cut down on saturated fats, increasing omega-3 fatty acids found in various fish, flaxseed oil and grapeseed oil. Via tincture or pill, mushroom Cordyceps boost good HDL cholesterol while reducing bad LDL. Before taking garlic, always consult you physician beforehand if you take the blood-thinning drug Coumadin.

Chronic Fatigue (Immune Dysfunction)

Epsetin-Barr Syndrome / Post Viral Fatigue Syndrome (PVFS)
Also see Thyroid Imbalance, Adrenal Imbalance, Hypoglycemia, Fibromyalgia, Energy Enhancement

The adrenal gland becomes exhausted from overuse, resulting in severe overall body exhaustion commonly called "chronic fatigue syndrome," or CFS. The usual causes are viruses such as Epstein-Barr virus and herpes virus 6, stress and excessive stimulants like caffeine. Never simple to diagnose, attempts to treat, chronic fatigue, Epstein-Barr Syndrome and Post Viral Fatigue Syndrome can also result from low blood pressure, immune system disorders, Lyme disease, viruses and systemic Candidiasis.

The lymph nodes often become tender, while other symptoms can include decreased sex drive, depression, mental cloudiness or memory loss, insufficient energy to perform normal tasks, and chronic fatigue lasting at least six months even amid continual rest and sleep. Mood swings can be just as disturbing as headaches and a disruption in sleep patterns.

Chronic Fatigue Causes

Low blood pressure is sometimes a suspected factor. Also, as previously mentioned, human herpes virus 6 and Epstein-Barr virus are often involved in chronic fatigue syndrome. Living a stressful life and excessive coffee sometimes trigger adrenal exhaustion that generates the severe fatigue. Some people suffering CFS have excessive amounts of candida albicans, a yeast usually found in healthful amounts within the bodies of most people.

Additional Considerations

In cases where health professionals initially fail to identify one of the above factors as the specific or likely causes, these specialists sometimes consider psychological or emotional causes as a likely factor. Here the suspected conditions might include depression, events that shock or traumatize the psyche or a chronic feeling of hopelessness. Also, physicians sometimes misdiagnose CFS, mistakenly listing the condition as Lyme disease. So, these may be co-infections occurring together.

Chronic Fatigue Treatments

Most important, you should support the adrenal glands, which trigger CFS when they become exhausted. (Visit the Adrenal Imbalance section of this guide for these specifics.) Use food therapies and antiviral herbs when a virus has caused these conditions. Excellent herbs include garlic extract, macà root, St. John's wort, and cat's claw. To treat, balance and augment low blood pressure, eat antioxidant-rich foods while taking iron supplements. Crops rich in bioflavonoid help, particularly bilberry, hawthorn root, gotu kola, green tea and red grapes. High-dose Vitamin C infusions may be helpful as well.

Cirrhosis

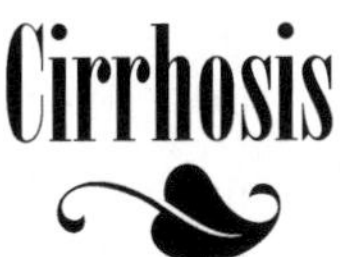

Also see Liver and Gallbladder Health, Inflammation

Adverse lifestyle choices and poor diets can lead to inflammation and scarring of the liver, "cirrhosis" that often generates severe health problems and even death. The condition sometimes builds gradually, promoting the development of long-term health problems that usually erupt before cirrhosis is finally diagnosed.

Particularly during the early stages of development, the symptoms can include itching, fever, indigestion, fatigue, constipation, altered stool color and diarrhea. More severe symptoms in later stages include pain, vomiting blood, easy bruising, and abdominal swelling and sometimes throughout the entire body—conditions that occasionally lead to comas, multiple organ failure or death.

Cirrhosis Causes

Alcoholism, drugs, exposure to toxins from the environment, Hepatitis B and C and from infections are among the most prevalent factors triggering cirrhosis.

Additional Considerations

Some patients have benefited from alternative remedies or treatments including Traditional Chinese Medicine and acupuncture.

Cirrhosis Treatments

Avoid alcohol, toxins or unnecessary use of harmful drugs, i.e. Tylenol, NSAIDS—even ignoring certain instances where physicians had previously prescribed the pharmaceuticals.

On the positive side, the liver is the body's only primary organ that can regenerate or regain healthful attributes even among adults well past puberty. So, eat natural foods without additives, and also take supplements or foods likely to help detoxify the body. These include raw liver tablets, lipoic acid, vitamins E and C, plus Vitamin B complex along with the amino acids L-arginine, L-glutathione, L-cysteine, milk thistle, and selenium.

Eat plenty of whole and organic foods like rice, soy or goat milk, seeds, green leafy vegetables, beans and nuts. Use flaxseed oil or olive oil rather than cold-processed oils, and avoid saturated or processed fats. Additional help comes from foods containing potassium and amino acids. Good sources include brewer's yeast, nuts, molasses, seeds, dulse, bananas, wheat bran, raisins and rice.

Meantime, avoid animal proteins that can cause liver stress or damage, particularly uncooked or raw fish. Enjoy "super-foods" loaded with green natural substances, or use "juice therapy"—particularly from apples—to detoxify the liver and the body. Always test your thyroid and adrenal function.

Cold Intolerance

Shivers, Cold Sensitivity, Chills

Also see Thyroid Imbalance, Energy Imbalance

Not to be confused with the "common cold," the term "cold intolerance" refers to conditions where a person feels a need to wear coats and sweaters—even while most other people feel comfortable amid similar environmental conditions.

Cold Intolerance Causes

Those experiencing such chills and shivering often lack adequate nutrition that would be necessary in order to avoid feeling unnecessarily uncomfortable amid mildly chilly environments.. Besides a lack of adequate protein, imbalances in the thyroid or adrenal system, and low blood pressure, adverse health conditions also can include chronic respiratory conditions, anorexia and insufficient levels of vital nutrients like iron or B vitamins.

Cold Intolerance Treatments

Load up on amino acids, protein, Vitamin C and liquid B-complex while increasing exercise. Significantly boost natural foods, avoid processed foods and add plenty of spices to your meals to increase the heart rate—particularly red pepper, curry, cayenne and turmeric. Get more help from yarrow, chamomile, boneset and ginger. Cayenne also improves circulation while energizing digestion. Run thyroid and adreneal tests.

Colds

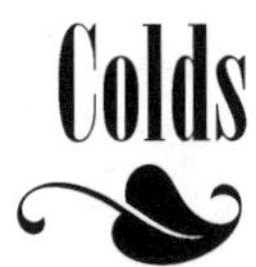

Also see Sore Throat, Infection (Bacterial), Infection (Viral)

That age-old saying still rings true, that indeed there "is no cure for the common cold." Thankfully, various natural remedies effectively eliminate or lessen symptoms, while also sometimes cutting the time that the person suffers.

Cold Causes

People catch colds in two ways, either exposure to viruses or becoming "run down." These conditions easily spread among people, particularly in unclean environments where bacteria or viruses thrive. Shaking hands or touching doorknobs are just as problematic as sneezes and coughs.

The dangerous viruses or bacteria usually enter people via the mouth, throat or nasal passages. The invaders begin attacking the nasal passages and throat, spreading to mucus membranes in the lungs—reaching the point where stopping symptoms becomes difficult.

Cold Prevention and Treatments

Fortify immunity with vegetable and fruit antioxidants, plus olive oil extract, colloidal silver, colostrum, Spirulina and Vitamin C—an essential vitamin particularly helpful in preventing colds amid chilly weather, when Echinacea with goldenseal also help.

Right when your throat first feels irritated or itchy, use a hand-held cold-killing throat spray containing antibacterial or antiviral grapefruit seed extract, propolis or tea tree oil and liquid Echinacea or liquid Saint John's wort. Use an eye-dropper if you don't have a spray tincture bottle.

Among other remedies sometimes recommended at the first sign of a cold: three times daily put a few drops in each ear of 3-percent hydrogen peroxide; and apply pomegranate topically to the throat as an antiviral. Colloidal silver or oregano sprays are also helpful.

Attack Existing Colds

Homeopaths and other practitioners of natural medicines have a cadre of formidable treatments for treating current colds. Among strategies:

Bacterial colds: These afflictions generating extremely runny noses require a little food added with 50 milligrams of picolinated zinc along with 100,000 IU of Vitamin A. Pregnant women or those who may become pregnant should avoid this level of the vitamin. Zinc helps by sharply boosting T-cells that fight infection, boosting the immune system while killing cold-causing bacteria. At least one study has indicated that zinc can cut the duration of cold symptoms and coughs by half, reducing mucus discharge by nearly one third.

Viral colds: When fevers accompany symptoms, take three grams of Vitamin C followed by one gram hourly until the fever breaks. Diarrhea sometimes occurs among patients who rarely or never take Vitamin C. Add L-lysine, colostrum and olive leaf extract.

Traditional Chinese Medicine: Ginger can snap a common cold when taken at the first sign of a cold, using three or four pieces of this substance to make tea. Add honey for flavor and basil if fever occurs.

Additional remedies: Accelerate results with three or four garlic capsules; herbs like Echinacea—preferably with goldenseal—accompanied by thymus glandular can help; olive leaf extract can serve as an antioxidant; licorice lozenges can naturally suppress coughs; and one cup of olive oil mixed with one tablespoon of horseradish can reduce symptoms like achy muscles.

Colon and Intestinal Health

Bowel Health / Colon Cleanse / Colonics / Colon Therapy / Enema

Also see Liver and Gallbladder Health; irritable Bowel Syndrome; Digestion; Diarrhea; Constipation; Candida

Most Americans take little care of their colon and bowels,

leading to dietary and health problems. Literally hundreds of parasites clog and slow down the body's excretion—which in healthy conditions run with relative ease. Just some of the many negative symptoms range from back pain, liver disease and headaches to an increased risk of parasites, food sensitivities, allergies, constipation and slow bowels, colon disease and irritable bowel syndrome, sluggishness, fatigue and a lack of energy, illnesses caused by bacteria or viruses, and more cramping and pain during PMS.

Additional Considerations

People with certain conditions should avoid colon therapy such as enemas. This is particularly important for individuals with intestinal tumors, severe hemorrhoids, diverticulitis, ulcerative colitis or Crohn's Disease. Among people without such conditions, coffee used in colonics and enemas rejuvenates the colon lining, stimulating its functions—while also cleaning essential bile ducts between the liver and colon. Afterward, reintroduce liquid chlorophyll to energize, heal and soothe the colon. Some people perform enemas on themselves if embarrassed about having a technician handle the procedure.

Healthy Colon Treatments

The best and most natural ways to treat colon problems involve diet, often because poor eating habits or negative choices generate many adverse conditions. Effective remedies for most conditions entail avoiding red meat, sugars, starches, dairy products and saturated fats.

Among the most effective colon-boosting strategies are colonics and enemas to clean away several pounds of unhealthful bacteria in the colon, removing waste and intestinal parasites, thereby restoring bowels to their youthful conditions. Besides coffee, multi-ingredient substances often helpful in cleaning the colon during colon cleanses are garlic extract, ground black walnut shells or husks; slippery elm, wormwood, yellow dock, aloe juice, citric acid from grapefruit or lemon, and cayenne pepper. This along with a healthful diet can help stop flatulence—particularly fiber and raw foods such as cabbage, Brussels sprouts and broccoli. Also, reducing cholesterol intake minimizes or prevents the buildup of fats and proteins that might clog the colon and intestines.

In addition, take healthful probiotic foods that boost healthy bacteria throughout the body, particularly in the intestines. Regenerate friendly fauna and flora by taking probiotic flora loaded with bifidophilus and acidophilus following chemotherapy, taking antibiotics or a colon cleanse. Antibiotics kill both healthy and harmful bacteria, so probiotics become necessary during or after taking such medications.

Conjunctivitis

Also see Macular Degeneration, Cataracts

Often called "pink eye," conjunctivitis occurs when the normally white cornea portion of the eye becomes pink when the mucus membrane that lines the eyes and eyelids become irritated. Symptoms include: sensitivity to light; watery eyes; swelling around the eyes; or itching, pain or irritation of the eye. Following naps or sleep, the eyelids can stick together.

Conjunctivitis Causes

Besides poor nutrition, the leading causes are stress, allergies, and infections. Bacteria sometimes move from the hands to the eyes when rubbing the eyes too much. Various drugs can lead to vision problems and conjunctivitis, particularly steroids, antihistamines, tetracycline, Digoxin, Chlorpromazine, and contraceptives.

Additional Considerations

Reverse or prevent vision problems by regularly exercising your eyes. Continually relaxing and then refocusing each time often helps. Roll your eyes in circular motions at least three times daily, also reducing eyestrain by regularly blinking.

Conjunctivitis Treatments

Enhance liver function with Traditional Chinese Medicine herbs like Ginkgo biloba and ginseng, thereby correcting vision problems. Benefit from nutritional supplements containing taurine, zinc, zeaxthanin, Selenium, vitamins E, A and B complex, plus beta-carotene, flavonoid, and N-acetyl-cysteine. Avoid alcohol, fried or processed foods, and excess sugar. Eat fresh fruit and organic whole foods because a healthful diet plays an integral role in conjunctivitis treatment. Focus largely on high-antioxidant vegetables, particularly citrus fruit, cherries, mangoes, purple or red grapes, dark rich-colored berries and dark leafy vegetables. Benefit from the high carotenoid content of organic egg yolks. Use topical antibiotics if necessary.

Constipation

Slow Bowels / Laxatives / Lazy Bowel Syndrome / Irregularity / IBS

Also see Irritable Bowel Syndrome, Digestion, Colon and Intestinal Health

The inability to completely defecate or to evacuate the rectum constitutes the condition that most people call "constipation." More specifically, however, the condition usually occurs because the colon has become clogged, malfunctioning, loaded with poisons or sluggish. Overall this problem is so critical that some medical professionals insist that cleaning the colon is a vital factor in overall good health. In general people in good or even poor health should remove excess waste and toxins from their colons—often deemed the fastest way to restore good health and "cure" disease.

But why—specifically—is cleaning the colon so important? Well, a clogged bowel impedes the body's—and the digestive system's—ability to process and to assimilate and process vital, essential and healthful nutrients. Homeopaths have identified a seemingly endless list of ailments and diseases that could be corrected or avoided by getting and maintaining a clean colon. A clogged colon can generate harmful or even severe problems with immune function, fertility, cholesterol, blood sugar, blood pressure, the heart, prostate, kidney and excessive body weight.

Compounding these dangers or problems, the colon is extremely large in comparison to the overall body while coming in close contact with all vital organs except the brain. This positioning becomes doubly dangerous, because it also makes critical contact with nerves and blood vessels throughout the abdominal area. As a result, constipation can cause the colon to suffer hernias or swelling.

Constipation Causes

A radical or sudden change in diet such as when traveling to a foreign country can be just as dangerous in disrupting colon function as medications, thyroid imbalance and intestinal disorders. People who fail to exercise or who move their bodies hardly at all, thereby engaging in a "sedentary lifestyle," increase their risk of problematic constipation. All narcotics used as medicine to control pain cause constipation to some degree.

Additional Considerations

While suffering from constipation, avoid over-the-counter laxatives that sometimes contain aloin, belladonna, strychnine or other poisons. In addition, cleansing the bowel is often advisable as a first-round measure when initially experiencing symptoms of various ailments or physical problems. Clearing the body of harmful toxins or other dangerous substances corrects and prevents many types of health problems. But when cleansing the body of toxins, be sure to effectively complete the process. Otherwise, the body might reabsorb the toxins, especially if the colon is not emptied during the overall bodily cleansing or "detoxification" effort.

Constipation Treatment

People who suffer constipation but who lack known medical issues should eat fibrous foods and drink lots of water. For people in this category, healthful amounts of Vitamin C and natural herbal laxatives like psyllium seed often helps. Eat plenty of fruit and vegetables, avoiding animal products like red meat and dairy.

Colonics help clean the colon, particularly when using natural substances that clear toxins from the colon. These include peppermint leaf, psyllium seed, slippery elm bark and marshmallow root.

Numerous natural substances also relieve constipation. A gentle but powerful way to restore regularity comes from cascara sagrada, an Amazon tree bark. Although this substance is considered both gentle and powerful, stop taking it as soon as bowel movements resume a regular pattern. The many other effective natural substances include ginger rhizomes, curacao, cape aloe leaf, senna leaves and pods, hobeero pepper, barberry root bark, and magnesium cytrate.

Corns

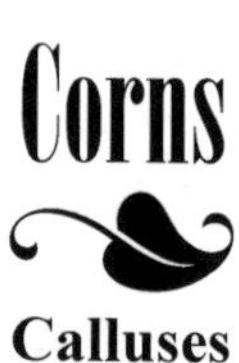

Calluses

The painful hard fleshy knots or wart-like bumps around or on the toes are commonly called "corns." Looking as if warts or infected calluses, corns sometimes become irritated or swollen—extremely painful when touched. Many medical professionals prefer to use sharp instruments to cut away these growths.

Corns Causes

Incorrect shoe sizes and high heels get much of the blame,

causing unnatural or irritating rubbing that generates the bumps. Infected calluses or warts sometimes cause corns. Walking in an awkward manner or with an unnatural gait sometimes generates the condition in people with knee or hip arthritis, or injuries.

Additional Considerations

Taken orally and topically, Vitamin A and Vitamin E nutritional supplements can help relieve symptoms. Wear clean socks and buy well-fitted shoes.

Corns Treatments

Relieve pain in the infected area with verucas essential oil or lemon, among other aromatherapy treatments. Three times daily, use anti-inflammatory agents and soften tissue by topically applying herbs like calendula petals and flower essence including arnica, and Rescue Remedy Cream. Hot water or ice can help vary temperatures in hydrotherapy strategies. Additionally, professional chiropractors, osteopaths or podiatrists can evaluate your bodily gait, to determine if you walk in a natural manner or in a way that causes irritation and rubbing that generates corns.

Cough

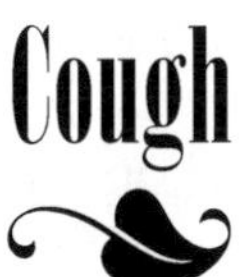

Also see colds

The body naturally reacts while coughing as a protective measure when infections, viruses or other health problems block air passages or the trachea. Mucus from the lungs or nasal passages or excess phlegm builds when a cold generates such symptoms. Viruses or bacteria generate the mucus buildup when these invaders attack the mucus membranes. This, in turn, generates sneezing or coughing as the invaders strive to spread to more people. In cases where viruses and bacteria are not involved, asthma, GERD, nasal problems or smoking sometimes generate chronic coughing—which can indicate serious diseases or infections including lung cancer, pneumonia or tuberculosis.

Additional Considerations

Positive results sometime emerge by orally taking a combination of licorice, slippery seed elm, ground apricot seed and ground perilla seed. Some homeopaths recommend taking up to 100,000 IU of Vitamin A daily until coughing dissipates. However, pregnant women and women who might become pregnant should avoid high levels of Vitamin A. At least one study has indicated that 25 milligrams of zinc taken daily can reduce by at least one-half the duration of coughing.

Cough Treatments

No single, universal, "catch-all" treatment or cure exists for coughs, because a wide variety of potential causes exist. So, rather than concentrate on the cause, in most cases medical professionals concentrate on curing or eliminating this symptom. Never eat foods that stimulate mucus, particularly sugar, dairy or starches.

People suffering coughs benefit from formidable "super foods," powders or mixes comprised primarily of health-enhancing corps including spinach, dandelion greens, kale, bee pollen and Spirulina. To fortify the immune system by battling cough-inducing pathogens, use clove, ginger, cayenne and cinnamon to reduce mucus.

Via room diffusers or steam humidifiers, use rosemary, pine, chamomile, peppermint, myrrh and eucalyptus. For coughs from allergies or colds, gargle with warm or "safely hot" sea salt water. As a gargle, use clove, turmeric, ginger, cinnamon or cayenne to reduce mucus.

Cysts

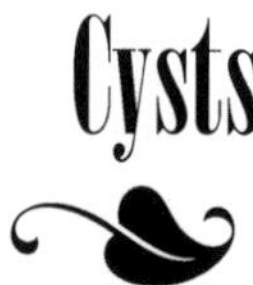

Also see Antiviral, Antibacterial, Anti-Inflammatory, Abscesses

Cysts appear on or inside the body in many forms, some irritating or unattractive or even dangerously big. These unwanted growths are mostly harmless, benign and non-cancerous. Common locations include the breasts, vagina, near vital glands or joints such as the knees or wrists, and at the neck or upper back.

Fluid under the skin gets trapped and accumulates, eventually forming cysts. Broken cysts usually cause pain. Vaginal cysts sometimes get infected or irritated, particularly during or after sexual activity.

Most cysts disappear naturally after a period of days, weeks, months or even years. Particularly with the help or guidance of a medical professional, patients can usually force cysts to dissipate. People should rely on a medical professional to drain large cysts to prevent abcesses.

Additional Considerations

People with cysts in on their breasts should avoid caffeine, a known cause of lumps or cysts in the breasts—particularly following menopause. Cysts of the cervix or ovaries usually disappear naturally, but visit a health care professional if they become large.

Cyst Treatments

Antibacterial and antiviral topical extracts can be effective in treating infections. Use ice packs to slow growth and moderate the pain of cysts in t he vagina or joints. Blood-thinning Vitamin E often proves an effective cyst-removal or prevention remedy, particularly when administered for six-month periods in high doses of 800-1,600 IU in a dry or succinate form. Reduce the dosage to 200-400 IU daily after the cyst disappears. For best results use tocotrienols. Rotate them to prevent the body from becoming overly accustomed to the same product.

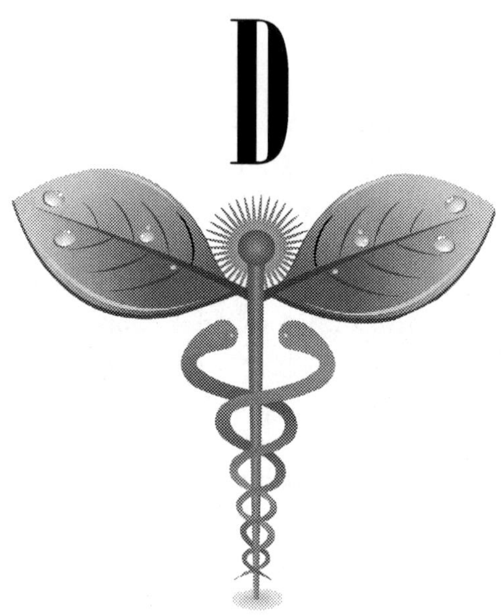
D

Dandruff

Seborrheic Dermatitis / Dry Scalp / Psoriasis

Also see Skin Health

While dandruff can damage a person's self-esteem, the condition is not a health threat. Even among healthy people the scalp skin dies and flakes away, naturally replaced by new skin. Dandruff occurs when this skin-cell replacement process accelerates. The shoulders and hair become littered with unsightly white flakes. Some dandruff types are itchy accompanied by scalp irritation.

Dandruff Causes

Although bacteria or fungus are usually to blame for scalp infections, various types of this condition have different causes. Physicians blame most dandruff cases on the Pityrosporum ovale fungus, naturally occurring in most people. This usually generates a non-itchy form of dandruff. Stress and chilly air are blamed for aggravating another form of dandruff called "seborrheic dermatitis," which can cause flakiness or redness even around the nose or eyebrows and hairline.

Physicians blame some instances of dandruff on anxiety, emotional stress that can damage the skin or scalp—worsening what otherwise would be a natural, barely noticed condition. Also, an unwanted health condition called "psoriasis," a difficult-to-diagnose mild autoimmune disorder sometimes causes skin problems including dandruff. (See the section on Autoimmune Disorders.) Contrary to popular belief, most people who suffer dandruff have oily rather than dry scalps—topically infected by fungus. Reduce the flakes by killing the fungus in a skin-drying process. This robs the fungus of a moist environment that it needs to survive.

Dandruff Treatments

Reduce or avoid antihistamines, which can exacerbate dandruff—particularly instances caused by seborrheic dermatitis. Numerous herbs effectively battle bacteria and fungus that trigger dermatitis. Besides Saint John's wort, apple cider vinegar baths and rinses are sometimes deemed as dermatitis and dandruff cures. Topically apply tea tree oil and oregano oil for additional results.

B-complex vitamins and Vitamin A at 25,000 IU battle dermatitis, and zinc sometimes reduces dandruff. Vitamin E and selenium supplements improve the skin's overall health. You also can topically apply selenium.

Homeopaths have developed a formidable herbal cure. Mix lavender, coltsfoot, rosemary, dandelion root, chamomile, horsetail, burdock root, and chaparral with two parts nettle. Then use a saucepan to boil enough water to rinse your hair. After removing the pan from the heat, let the water cool beginning when you sprinkle the herbs on top. Be sure to avoid sprinkling the herbs while boiling. Shampoo your hair as you normally do, before pouring the herb decoction over your head. Some people use the herb decoction daily rather than shampoo, which dries the hair.

Dehydration

Failing to drink adequate amounts of pure water can lead to dehydration, deemed a factor in a variety of serious health conditions. These include ulcers, prostate problems, worsening vision, kidney failure, kidney stones and Alzheimer's Disease.

Additional Considerations

People can become dehydrated in dry or humid environments. Severe instances of dehydration sometimes require intravenous hydration, often called "IVs."

Dehydration Causes

Besides failing to drink enough liquids, dehydration can be caused by excessive sweating or overexertion. Drinking too much alcohol or caffeine also can rob the body of adequate levels of vital moisture. So, drink additional water if you use these. Overweight people also should drink lots of water, particularly if exerting themselves.

Get checked for diabetes if you're always thirsty. The many dehydration symptoms include lethargy, nausea, edema, toxemia, dry skin, dry mouths, headaches and dizziness. Additional problems involve nausea, constipation, dark urine, infrequent urination, low blood pressure, an overly acidic body, achy joints—particularly in the big toe, and premature aging signs like wrinkles, a listless tone and dark circles under the eyes.

Dehydration Treatments and Cures

Drink at least eight to ten 8-ounce glasses of pure water daily. Water generates best results, although other non-alcoholic and non-caffeine drinks can re-hydrate the body, particularly coconut water or carbon activated water. To make the body quickly absorb water, add a tablespoon of sugar and a few pinches of salt to a quart.

Depression

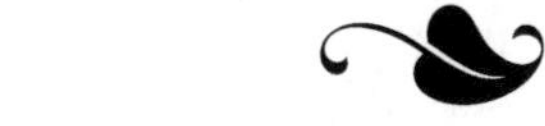

Post Partum Depression / SAD / Bipolar Disorder / Manic Depression

Almost every person suffers from depression at some point in life. Most of the time, the depression subsides after being triggered by a specific cause or a mentally disturbing event. Yet depression sometimes becomes long-term, more in women than men. Sometimes leading to illness, substance abuse or other problems, long-term depression impacts the person's ability to cope or to function normally within society.

Some people suffering depression lose or gain lots of weight. Depressed individuals suffer everything from: an inability to make decisions, lacking concentration or focus; a lack of mental or physical energy; suicidal thoughts; substance abuse; alcoholism; nervous energy; and continual feelings of shame, hopelessness, guilt, failure, a low self image, and low libido.

Types of Depression

Researchers have identified numerous specific types of depression. Entire books have been written on each specific form. Here is a brief summary:

Chronic Depression: Either intense or mild, this long-term variety lasts four months or more. "Suicidal ideation"—an unusual preoccupation with suicide—is not uncommon in this condition.

Transitory Depression: Sudden or depressing events cause this condition, such as the sudden death of a loved one or the breakup of a relationship. Although sometimes intense, this type of depression usually subsides or disappears within several months.

Post Traumatic Stress Disorder: Auto accidents or other traumatic events including war battles ignite this depression—which also can occur after "positive" traumatic events such as a major musical or acting performance by the person.

Post Partum Depression: This happens when women suffer depression after childbirth.

Seasonal Depression: This usually occurs during the winter, called SAD—season adaptive depression—when there is less sunlight and weather becomes colder and perhaps "dreary" in the mind of the person.

Manic Depression / Bipolar Disorder: The person experiences significant mood swings, usually morbidly depressed or overly positive. Severe forms usually result in a bipolar diagnosis. Hypersexual behavior may be a manifestation of a hyper-manic state.

Depression Causes

A vast array of factors can generate depression, sometimes involving repressed emotions, memories or events. Ultimately, only a few primary causes exist:

Chemicals: A chemical imbalance occurs within the body, disrupting the brain and nervous system neurotransmitters, or causing hormonal imbalances. Despite recent overall advances in modern medicine and treatment as a whole, researchers remain unsure whether these imbalances are caused by depression, or if they're symptoms.

Emotional and Mental: In adults and children, emotional and physical abuse, and emotional trauma, can cause depression. Triggering events include financial woes, death of a loved one, traumatic occurrences or relationship problems. Some people suffer depression when they "repress" or fail to express their emotions.

Depression Treatments

Homeopaths can administer a variety of remedies often deemed effective in naturally treating specific types of depression.

Vitamins and Supplements: Rather than risk addiction and bodily damage caused by prescription antidepressants, strive to benefit from natural substances administered as vitamins or supplements. Lots of patients report feeling incredible within days after starting to take nutritional formulas targeting depression. Natural substances often deemed effective include St. John's wort, dehydroepiandrosterone (DHEA), glutamic acid or glutamine powder, choline, phosphatidlyserine, tyrosine, 5HTP, theanine, phenylalanine, and S-adenosyl-methionine (SAM-E). **Caution**: *Avoid taking nutritional supplements until at least six weeks after stopping the antidepressant monoamine oxidase inhibitor or MAOI—which takes at least a month and a half to naturally leave the body. While taking MAOI, patients also must follow the orders of doctors or pharmacists to avoid certain foods or drinks including wines, liquors and non-alcoholic beers that may contain tyramine—an amino acid that adversely reacts with DHEA.*

Food: Eat fruit, especially crops like mangoes or apples that fortify the body with vitamins and antioxidants. Pure cocoa and dark chocolates can help improve a person's mood thanks to specific nutrients that address depression—particularly theabroma, a methyl-xanthine. Avoid alcohol, which prevents the brain from receiving essential omega-3 fatty acids. Also steer clear of processed, starchy, sugary, high-fructose foods, and dairy.

Lifestyle: Depression can subside or disappear at least somewhat when the circulatory and lymphatic systems get stimulated by exercise. Body movements generated by exercise make the body produce two feel-good brain chemicals, endorphins and serotonin. Relaxing baths and saunas, particularly with healing aromas and herbs, can help the mind relax.

Essential Oils and Herbs: Specific natural herbs serve as excellent antidepressants, particularly pine, rosemary, mint, geranium, rose and bergamot oils.

Additional Considerations

The adrenal steroid, sometimes called DHEA, impacts the vital brain cell membranes—particularly the fluidity within that region. This attribute makes DHEA an important option in attempting to stabilize mood swings associated with bipolar disorder and lessening depression. Some doctors believe DHEA has an effectiveness similar to lithium, but without the potentially problematic side effects. Homeopaths sometimes recommend 10-25 mg of DHEA as a supplement at bedtime.

Diabetes

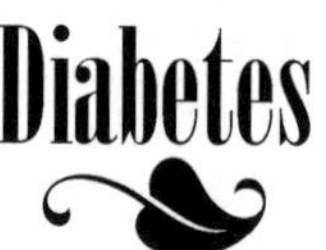

High Blood Sugar / Diabetes Mellitus

Also see Thyroid Imbalance, Hypoglycemia, Cardiovascular Health, High Blood Pressure

Relatively common in the U.S.A., diabetes features dangerously high blood sugar usually sparked by excessive amounts of carbohydrates and sugars. Too much caffeine indirectly contributes to the problem by hampering thyroid function and creating hormonal imbalances that trigger diabetes. This is often triggered by cancer of the pancreas or adrenal glands.

Besides thirst and frequent urination, common symptoms include headaches, erectile dysfunction, blurred vision, fatigue, and weight loss as appetite increases.

Diabetes Causes

Everything comes down to the fact that too much sugar or glucose in the blood causes diabetes. This condition generates an issue with insulin, which carries blood sugar to cells throughout the body. When blood sugar levels increase to excessive levels, the body responds with insulin resistance—pushing up glucose levels dangerously high. Eating too much sugar, especially fructose, is another cause. Among primary diabetes causes:

Obesity: Excessive body weight can generate hormonal and insulin issues, worsening or causing diabetes.

Diet: Excessive caffeine, fat and sugar are usually to blame.

Poor liver health: Damaged livers prevent or hinder the body's ability to process sugars and to cleanse the blood, resulting in diabetes.

Chronic steroid use: Using these potentially dangerous drugs wrecks or changes body chemistry, worsening or causing diabetes.

Thyroid imbalance: An adverse response to insulin can result from thyroid or adrenal problems that generate hormonal imbalances, contributing to or causing diabetes.

Diabetes Treatments

Right after an initial diagnosis of diabetes, modify or correct your diet with the professional assistance of a dietitian or other medical professional. Among natural strategies:

Clean: People craving sweets sometimes have parasites in their systems while lacking sufficient protein. After the colon and liver get cleaned the body benefits from an increased ability to absorb vital nutrients.

Boost immunity: Take healthful amounts of multivitamins and particularly antioxidants that help address or prevent free radical problems that generate some of the worst outcomes—including blindness, or limb amputation.

Avoid sugars: Never eat sugary products or substances, including malt, lactose-filled dairy products; sorbitol, glucose, corn starch, dextrose, fructose from fruit or corn syrup; or sucrose derived from maple cane or sugar.

Enjoy low-glycemic foods: These healthy foods and crops lower glycemic levels, particularly raw rather than cooked foods. Healthy options include yams, potatoes, green leafy vegetables, chicken, legumes, nuts, whole grain breads and fish.

Herbs: The various herbs helpful in lowering blood sugar include olive leaves, genugreek, ginseng, garlic and bilberry. Get additional help from supplements of bitter lemon, chromium, cinnamon, and vanadium. Supplements also should include Vitamin E, which prevents the type of yeast infections diabetics are prone to suffer.

Carbohydrates and Starches: Glucose that worsens or generates diabetes is created when the body converts starches from carbohydrates. Besides sugar, simple carbohydrates include honey, dairy products, fruit juice and fruit. Processed meat, peanut butter, cheese and soybean oil create similar dangers, so avoid them as well. Minimize your intake of complex carbohydrates, particularly fibrous vegetables like eggplant and squash, pasta, breads, beans, and grains. Although whole wheat is better than processed grain-based products, enjoy the benefit more by instead taking natural grains like barley, rye, bran and oats.

Additional Considerations

Garlic benefits cardiovascular health, making this an important food or supplement for diabetics because such individuals are prone to heart disease. Some homeopaths recommend B-complex vitamins to prevent diabetic neuropathy and poor circulation, a precursor to limb amputation.

Additional Diet and Supplement Tips

Control blood sugar by taking oxygen-rich aloe vera juice, derived from the inside of the plant with the toxic outer skin removed. To block tongue receptors that register sweetness and thereby reduce cravings for such foods, chew the gymnema sylvestre or gurmar leaf hailed in India as "the poor man's insulin." This gives sweets a bland, displeasing cardboard taste, eliminating the cravings or desire for such food. For best results, chew gurmar daily for at least six weeks.

A natural plant used in Japan for 1,000 years, konjac-mannan, lowers blood sugar. You can also purify the blood and battle antioxidants with lipoic acids (LA) or alpha-lipoic acid. Beneficial to diabetes patients and available as supplements without prescription, the biological properties of LA correct the body's response to insulin sensitivity, while improving how glucose responds to insulin. Great food sources for LA include Brussels sprouts, tomatoes, broccoli and spinach.

Diarrhea

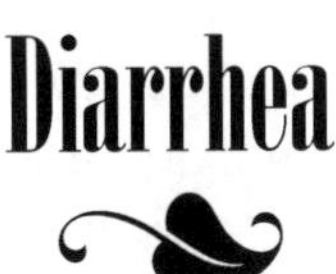

Also see Colon and Intestinal Health

"What's causing this?" Many people immediately ask themselves as the first sign of diarrhea. This symptom or condition usually stems from food allergies or an illness like the flu, passing through the body within several days. Yet diarrhea occasionally signals an underlying health problem, sometimes significant. Seek medical attention if diarrhea causes significant weight loss or persists at least ten days.

Diarrhea Causes

To clearly understand what causes diarrhea, patients first need to know that this condition occurs when the colon fails to function properly—usually due to disease, infection, irritations or inflammation.

Disease: Serious ailments or diseases trigger diarrhea. Culprits include radiation sickness, Crohn's disease, amebic dysentery, typhoid fever and food poisoning from Shigella bacteria, cholera, staphylococcus bacteria or cholera and Norwalk virus, and certain parasites.

Vitamin C: Most people suffer diarrhea after taking too much Vitamin C, so reduce your intake of this nutrient if the colon problem occurs amid a mega-dosing regimen of this substance. Excessive magnesium also triggers diarrhea.

Parasites: Severe diarrhea requires medical attention when caused by parasites that the person comes into contact with by eating undercooked meat, coming into contact with the invaders while traveling or touching animals or unsanitary conditions. Take probiotics after any treatment that uses antiboitics.

Dairy products: Rather than manifesting as hives or other common allergy symptoms, some people adverse to dairy products respond with diarrhea. Avoid dairy products for at least two weeks if you suffer chronic diarrhea. Then, if the problem persists, you can rule out dairy allergies as a possible cause.

Food reactions: The body sometimes reacts adversely to certain food, depending on the person's individualized sensitivity to certain meals, crops or beverages. Some people, for instance, cannot tolerate spicy food while others need to avoid beer. When this happens the body uses diarrhea to rid itself of "biologically perceived" or unwanted toxins. Allergic reactions to lactose sugar and gluten become more prevalent with aging.

Viruses: Both mild and severe viral infections can cause diarrhea.

Diarrhea Treatments

Always treat the cause of diarrhea rater than merely the symptom. Yet you should always take certain measures, whatever the cause. Avoid beverages and foods that have been fermented, processed foods, alcohol, dairy and caffeine. With equal dedication, take: antiviral, antibacterial and antifungal herbs such as Saint John's wort, barberry root, or the extracts of green tea, garlic or oregano; plenty of nutrient-rich food supplements; probiotic cultures to address fungus even if fungal infections did not cause your diarrhea; and nutrient-rich supplements to restore minerals and vitamins that diarrhea removed from the body.

Additional Considerations

Watch for potentially catastrophic or even life-threatening dehydration if diarrhea is severe. Get immediate medical attention in such instances, drink lots of pure water, and also green tea to fight bacteria. Also visit a doctor when a child suffers diarrhea more than two days. Restore minerals and lost vitamins with a teaspoon of bee pollen. Eliminate symptoms with fibrous foods like bran or wheat germ, bananas and plain yogurt. Except for bananas, never use flavoring or sugar. Hydrate the body via IV if necessary.

Herbalists sometimes recommend goldenseal or grapefruit seed extract. Colloidal silver is often effective battling infections that cause diarrhea, going to the colon to kill "bad bacteria." This proves formidable for people with compromised or weakened immune symptoms hampered by medical conditions or diseases such as AIDS.

For instance, the immune systems of healthy people usually can effectively fight potentially dangerous cryptosporidium parasites. But those invaders can cause life-threatening diarrhea among people with weakened immune systems. Use barberry root to effectively treat virus-caused diarrhea, while hampering the ability to E. coli virus to flourish within the colon.

Digestion

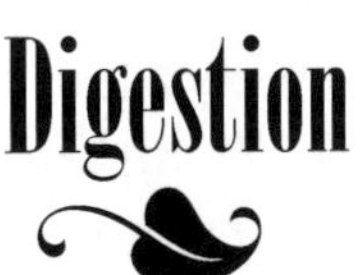

Indigestion / Digestive Cramps

Also see Liver and Gallbladder Health, Flatulence, Heartburn

Like all other animals including plants, microorganisms and mammals, humans convert formerly living things through a digestion process needed to generate energy necessary for sustaining life. The digestion process in humans begins with chewing, before the stomach and intestines break down the food further in a chemical process.

People are "omnivores," animals that have slow digestive systems taking at least 24 hours to complete after eating plants. Another type of animal, carnivores, have bodies that process food into energy fast, in as little as two hours. This prevents meat from sitting in the digestive tracts of such animals.

Unlike all other herbivores, people are the only such animals that eat meat. In humans this can lead to poor digestion, plus a variety of other health problems ranging from fatigue and breathing problems to oily skin and acne.

Digestion Problem Causes

Numerous giant volumes could be compiled on the factors causing digestive problems in people. In summary, humans risk suffering digestive difficulties when eating too much fat, meat, sugar, protein and caffeine. An overall unhealthful diet, in conjunction with one or more of these factors, can trigger chemical imbalances, plus an unhealthy buildup of toxins and waste within the body.

Exacerbating these problems, some people suffer adverse food reactions generating indigestion, nausea or cramping. Additional problems stem from toxins within food and environmental toxins like heavy metals within the person's personal or work area.

Rather than leaving the body via the bowels, excess fat hampers functioning of the liver and gallbladder. Sugar harms the digestive system when stored as fat. Illness sometimes occurs because the human digestive system does a poor job processing meat, which often slows the intestines and bowels. Proteins derived from dairy and red meat also slow the digestive system, hampering the body's ability to metabolize nutrients. Worsening matters, caffeine slows digestion by generating adrenal hormones.

Digestive System Treatments

Everything hinges on diet. Healthful diets prevent or treat digestive problems, while eating "unhealthy food" causes such issues. So, avoid cheese, fried food, butter and other fatty selections. Far better choices encompass raw or lightly cooked vegetables, whole grains and rice. Never drink water during mealtime to refrain from diluting vital stomach acids when they're essential. Besides chewing well before swallowing, you also can boost digestion by eating oranges, apples and avocadoes.

Certain food combinations also can wreak havoc on digestion. Never eat fruit while also digesting animal proteins or carbohydrates. Avoid tomato sauces, greasy or oily foods and soft drinks. Instead, eat garlic and onions to aid digestion, but afterward you can employ an East India tradition—chewing fennel seeds or licorice to remove bad breath and to prevent flatulence.

Use activated carbon supplements to remedy digestive maladies like nausea, acid indigestion and heartburn. Follow a greasy meal with a cup of hot yerba mate or green tea to help digestion. Numerous natural digestive enzymes also can help, including protease, papain, and bromelain. Probiotics and enzymes help remove excess waste buildup from the digestive tract. Another good digestive enhancement is ginger, which also helps prevent nausea and vomiting.

Diverticulitis

Diverticulosis

Also see Irritable Bowel Syndrome, Diarrhea, Constipation, Colon and Intestinal Health

The typical American diet causes pouches or balloon-shaped sacks called "diverticulosis" to form on the intestinal walls, sometimes becoming painful and inflamed. People who eat only whole, natural foods including vegetables and fruit rarely suffer from this condition. Common symptoms include excessive gas, bloody, dark or mucus-filled stools, diarrhea, constipation, abdominal pain, and symptoms similar to appendicitis or irritable bowel syndrome.

Diverticulitis Causes

Health professionals blame poor diets for causing diverticulitis. Going for extended periods without eating healthful foods like fiber-rich meals, vegetables and fresh fruit lead to the condition. A sedentary lifestyle, drugs, food allergies and "leaky gut" syndrome also are among causes. A "leaky gut" often leads to severe health problems as food particles remain undigested while moving through the gastrointestinal tract.

Almost all antibiotics and drugs seemingly as harmless as aspirin can irritate and cause gastrointestinal disorders. Other potential offenders here include analgesic tablets, Voltaren, Prokine, Ecotrin and cuprimine.

Additional Considerations

Processes such as exercise, hyperthermia, and far infrared sauna treatments that induce sweat can help remove toxins from the body. This, in turn, minimizes the presence of viruses and bacteria, which die when body temperature increases above normal healthy levels.

Diverticulitis Treatments

Exercising generally improves bowel function. Also, physicians warn that smoking worsens diverticulitis, so stop or at least curtail that unhealthful habit. A highly organic diet rich in whole foods and fiber are necessary in preventing or reversing diverticulitis. First, never have coffee or alcohol, or foods likely to cause allergies including shell fish, wheat, dairy and soy, and also avoid sugars, refined carbohydrates and processed food.

Some homeopaths and dietitians recommend that attempts at herbal remedies should start with licorice root tea taken with

"Robert's Formula," a healthful combination of wild indigo, slippery elm, comfrey, poke root, Echinacea, marshmallow root, geranium, and goldenseal.

The best strategy also involves eating more steamed vegetables, cooked whole grains, easy-to-digest antioxidant vegetables and fruits, and free-range organic poultry and meat. For best results, avoid all meat for awhile, commencing as the diet change begins.

Colocynthis, bryonia and belladonna are among remedies prescribed by homeopaths. Nutritional supplements include probiotics like Bifidobacteria and acidophilus, plus Vitamin C and B-complex vitamins.

Dizziness

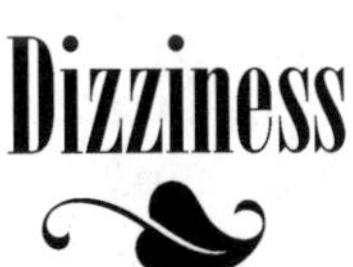

Vertigo / Disequilibrium

Also see Motion Sickness, Anemia, Anxiety

Some dizzy people feel as if falling or spinning, while others complain of feeling "off balance." An added complaint involves vertigo, sometimes associated with heights or emotional stress—often either objective vertigo when objects seem to spin all around, or subjective vertigo when the person feels as though she or he is spinning.

Severe vertigo can cause hearing loss or "tinnitus," ringing in the ears. Inner-ear problems cause what doctors call "true vertigo," sometimes also associated with the eyes, brain stem, cranial nerves or middle ear. Dizziness rarely involves symptoms often caused by vertigo such as severe sweating, vomiting or nausea—sometimes triggered by viral infections.

Dizziness Causes

Stress, anxiety, depression and fatigue, low blood pressure, or even low blood sugar levels are among frequent causes. Iron deficiencies or even adverse drug reactions cause such problems.

Other possible factors include: temporarily insufficient levels of blood in the brain, adrenal exhaustion from excessive stimulants, cerebellar tumors, head trauma, adrenal exhaustion, middle- and inner-ear diseases often associated with chronic sinusitis.

Dizziness Treatments

Avoid processed foods or meals loaded with unnatural preservatives. Gingko leaf extract and ginger can help. Reduce alcohol, caffeine and sugar, while maintaining blood sugar levels by eating small meals throughout the day. Potentially beneficial supplements include iron. When anemia is the cause homeopaths recommend iron-rich foods like dark green leafy vegetables, bee pollen, raw seeds, kale and spinach.

Get more nutrients from supplements rich in Vitamin E, niacin and B-complex vitamins. Non-traditional medicines like acupuncture sometimes help. Get additional assistance from Granataum, Convallaria, Gelsemium, Cocculus, and Phosphorus.

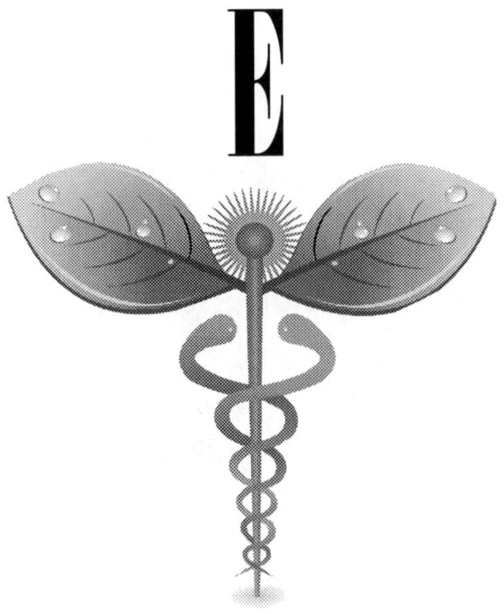
E

Ear Infection

Many people fail to realize that the primary culprit that sparks ear infections is merely "blowing your nose the wrong way." The other primary triggers are allergens, adverse reactions to milk, and water entering the ear canal. Rare instances result from surgical complications or congenital defects.

Healthy people have natural biological systems connecting their ears, throat, eyes and nose. Nasal passages are connected via Eustachian tube to each ear. Incorrectly blowing the nose can block these vital tubes. Avoid this problem by keeping the mouth open while simultaneously exhaling through both nostrils while blowing the nose. Exhaling through just one nostril while blowing the nose can push mucus into the Eustachian tube, usually on the other side of the head.

Water entering the ear passages can become trapped in the ear canal, creating a potential growth site for harmful fungi and bacteria. The typical symptoms of such infections are: hearing loss; yellow secretions from the ear; a chronically itchy ear canal; and pain in the inner, outer or middle ear.

Ear Infection Causes

Earwax sometimes fails to drain as it does naturally in healthy people. Flu and cold infections sometimes congest the middle ear, potentially leading to inflammation or hearing loss. Swimming in polluted water sometimes enables harmful bacteria to enter the ear canal.

Additional Considerations

Some children are prone to ear infections due to inadequate drainage systems within their mouths. Sadly, antibiotics occasionally prescribed to treat these problems sometimes destroy "friendly bacteria," thereby actually extending the duration of the problem. Painful chronic ear infections can occur as a result. So, avoid harmful, unnatural antibiotics—and instead use natural probiotics, silver, colostrum and olive leaf extracts.

Ear Infection Prevention and Treatments

Administered gently via ear-drops into the ear canal, natural products frequently used to treat ear infections include unscented warm garlic oil, diluted grapefruit seed extract, and apple cider vinegar. Also, remember that some people incorrectly use cotton swabs in failed efforts to remove earwax. Instead, the swabs push this substance deeper into the ear canal, causing a buildup that can lead to damage to the eardrums, infections and hearing loss. Instead, use a rubber ear bulb syringe purchased at a drugstore to gently rinse the ear with a 50-50 solution of water and hydrogen peroxide as a 3-percent solute.

Eczema

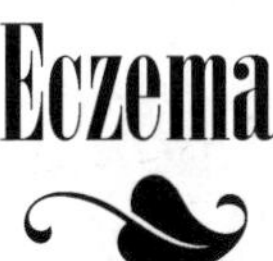

Dermatitis / Skin Rash

Also see Stress, Dandruff, Liver and Gallbladder Health

Cracking, dry or flaky skin, blistering, redness and itching are among bothersome symptoms of eczema. Called a form of dermatitis, this skin rash can appear almost anywhere on the body—often in areas where the skin folds on the face, buttocks and under the breasts.

Eczema Causes

Health professionals cite a variety of potential causes, usually ranging from iron deficiencies and poor diet to allergies and poor liver function or Vitamin B deficiencies.

Eczema Treatments

Avoid perfumes and only wear cotton clothes. Take iron

supplements if a deficiency in that element is deemed the cause. Work to alleviate stress if that's deemed a likely cause. (See the Stress section of this guide.) Mixing burdock root with figwort and nettles can address the stress factor.

Sometimes used topically as an antifungal or 1-percent hydrocortisone (OTC) used daily can emerge as effective until the eczema disappears. Non-flavored Listerine-brand mouthwash that lacks artificial sweeteners can be used to effectively wash the rash.

Positive results are possible from natural bifidophilus and acidophilus probiotics, plus natural substances like picolinated zinc, Vitamin E, B-complex vitamins, iodine seaweeds, copper and inositol.

To correct liver disorders that sometimes cause eczema, detoxify the liver and blood with burdock root, sometimes mixed with cleaves or red clover.

Edema

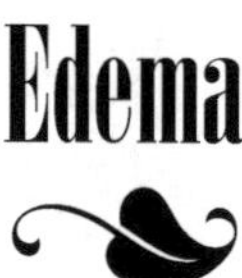

Swelling / Ascites

Also see Liver and Gallbladder Health, Cardiovascular Health

The excessive buildup of fluids within the body or lower extremities causes or is the result of edema, which can occur in the lower extremities, knees, feet, face and hands. Serious instances can involve swelling of the brain, leading to memory issues, headaches and even behavioral changes. Severe or extreme cases can lead to overall weight gain, a dangerous buildup of fluid in the lungs and a bloated abdomen.

Edema Causes

Infrequent instances strike people who fly in airplanes at low altitude for extended periods. Climate changes are also sometimes blamed. Health care professionals have pinpointed many edema cases to problems with the kidneys, liver and the cardiovascular system. Typical causes are the failure of the liver, kidney or heart.

Additional potential causes also include pelvis or groin tumors, hypothyroidism, Vitamin B deficiencies, and protein absorption issues.

Edema Treatments

Homeopaths often recommend dietary changes that usually minimize or reduce edema. Take carbon-activated water to hydrate the body. The best anti-edema foods have high water content, especially watermelon, potatoes, cabbage, citrus fruits, onion, beets, apples and cucumbers. Potassium-rich dandelion leaf and horse-chestnut seed extract are helpful herbal remedies.

Use hydrotherapy, far infrared radiation or massage to help detoxify the body. Just as important, avoid dairy products, fried food, salt, alcohol and caffeine, also steering clear of cured foods, white flower, sugar, processed grains, and meat. Instead, enjoy healthy, nutrient rich meals and supplements loaded with nutrition. Help sometimes comes from alfalfa tables and free-form amino acids. Effective anti-edema supplements include potassium, Vitamin C, Vitamin B6, B-complex vitamins, pantothetic acid, and low-sodium diets.

Energy Enhancement

Vitality / energy Drinks / Lethargy / Low energy / Stimulants
Also see Thyroid Imbalance, Adrenal Imbalance, Chronic Fatigue Syndrome, Hypoglycemia

Energetic, ambitious and creative people usually feel young and healthy. In fact, in the public mindset, high energy is usually associated with youthful individuals. More importantly, people of all ages need ample energy in mind and body in order to function in a healthful, vibrant manner.

As biological mechanisms for slow-burning our necessary "fuel"—food—humans need the best nutrition sources in order to remain alive and to thrive physically and mentally. When people feel lethargic or sluggish, they sometimes seek stimulants to boost or to enhance their personal energy levels. But what causes fatigue and what naturally reverses the condition?

Complex and even simple characteristics are involved. Our bodies require glucose derived from food to survive and to thrive. Transported via the blood, glucose is converted by our livers into storage glycogen needed by the cells to burn as fuel.

Low Energy Causes

Blood sugar provides the chemical energy that our bodies need. Yet potential problems can emerge if the digestive and insulin hormone transportation system go haywire. When the liver fails to efficiently convert glucose into glycogen excess sugars convert into fat. Breakdowns can occur in numerous phases of what otherwise would be a healthy energy-producing and energy-using process.

Potential problems can include everything from a low-energy or no-energy "crash" to a high nervous energy. Triggering factors or symptoms can include poor cellular health, low blood pressure, the low insulin levels of diabetes and the low blood sugar of hypoglycemia.

Medical professionals sometimes cite additional potential factors, particularly insufficient muscle mass, thyroid or adrenal imbalances and poor liver health.

Additional Considerations

Muscle and tissue energy comes mostly from glucose, with the best source as complex carbohydrates like beans, vegetables and grain. Normalize circulation with pure cocoa, also an ideal antioxidant that also improves mood. But avoid eating too much chocolate. Good non-caffeine natural energy boosters include: gensing; maca, a Peruvian root; suma—a South American root, and seaweed-based organic minerals.

Enhance Energy

Strive to live free of unnecessary emotional baggage or stress that can rob your psyche and ultimately the body of vital energy. Some people sense an unhealthful need to enhance their energy with caffeine or dangerous and highly addictive stimulant narcotics. Others strive to benefit from a much more preferable, natural and safe strategy employing healthy energy-boosting foods and supplements such as alpha lipoic acid, resveratrol and arginine.

The adaptogenic herb Schizandra berry used in Traditional Chinese Medicine can help boost energy and strength while balancing various bodily systems. Some Chinese herbalists believe the berry can increase life expectancy.

Amazingly, many people still need to learn that generally eating lower quantities of food—not more—actually increases the body's energy efficiency. For best results, strive to eat an ideal amount of fats, carbohydrates and proteins. Yet each person has unique, individual biological needs and challenges. So, employing a dietitian or homeopath is highly recommended to generate a diet plan best for your specific needs.

A person's energy level usually accelerates upon losing excess, unneeded body fat. Purify the body of toxins and excess roughage or waste that may be slowing your energy levels. Stay away from artificial energy sources such as EMG sources, X-ray, CAT scans and PET scans.

Minimize the intake of fructose derived from goods like syrup and fruit, converted only by the liver into energy—with all excess stored as fat within body tissue. So, avoid high-fructose corn syrup, a common juice additive.

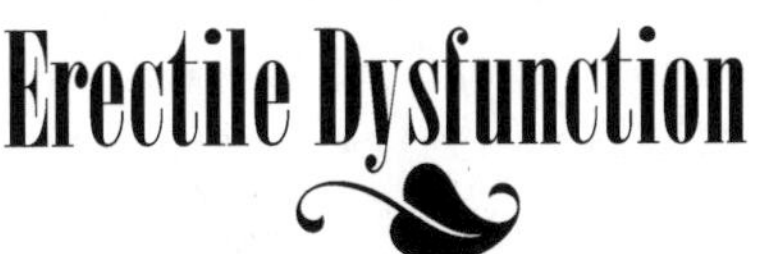

ED / Impotence

Also see Sexual Dysfunction, Prostate Health

Often called "ED," erectile dysfunction has boomed into a

multi-billion-dollar industry, particularly since the early 1990s. Yet many people fail to realize that whenever "unnatural" drugs are used dangerous long-term side effects can occur. Most ED products delivered to the public mindset strive to boost nitric oxide, a key biological mechanism in enabling men to have erections.

However, the same substance also has been blamed for creating inflammation in joints and body tissues. Inflammation can lead to serious health conditions including arthritis and even cancer, although there has been no proof that ED medications cause such diseases.

Erectile Dysfunction Causes

Prostate disorders and diabetes remain at or near the top of the list of causes. Medical experts also blame chronic fatigue syndrome and Lyme disease for low energy, even relatively mild neuro-emotional or psychological issues, hormonal, thyroid or adrenal imbalances, and pituitary issues. Other known or suspected causes include depression, peripheral arterial disease, anti-inflammatory medicines, toxins from foods and drugs, and sedentary lifestyles. Pharmaceuticals also are factors, particularly blood pressure medications, anti-psychotics, analgesics and anti-depressants.

Erectile Dysfunction Treatments

Since a huge portion of ED cases stem from vascular problems created by diabetes, men experiencing this problem should have their physician check them for this disease. Prostate issues also generate some erectile problems, so you should initially avoid ruling this out this as well. (See the sections on Diabetes and Prostate Health.) The popular ED drug Viagra was initially used to treat diabetes. Yet natural cures are far more preferable. Besides addressing the potential underlying causes of diabetes and prostate issues, a large selection of natural herbs can help. Among instances:

For those who prefer, rather than using herbs, or sometimes in combination with such natural substances, some men may benefit by using the mindful, meditative "tantric tradition." This strategy strives to control the body's natural energy flow, particularly involving the sexual organs. Occasionally, bio-identical testosterone cream is necessary to increase testosterone levels.

Natural foods like mangoes, bananas, cinnamon and peanuts can stimulate sex drive while enhancing performance. To improve circulation and thereby improve functions of the body's various sexual functions, the spices cayenne, curcumin, coriander, cinnamon and clove often help—primarily by increasing blood flow to the genitals.

Some men claim that various natural substances work as well as Viagra, while lacking the potentially harmful inflammation attributes of some pharmaceuticals. Substances known to generate nitric oxide while increasing blood flow to the penis include L-arginine, hailed as "the poor man's Viagra." Also try maca, yohimbe, tongkat ali, Rhodiola rosea, and horny goat extract (weed), DHEA, ginseng, sea buckhorn and mung bean sprout.

Picolinated zinc combined with Vitamin E or E-complex vitamins can intensify erections, while also increasing the potential arousal of women by increasing testosterone. Some men, particularly athletes, also take mushroom Cordyceps, a plant-based performance enhancer that boosts energy while intensifying erections.

F

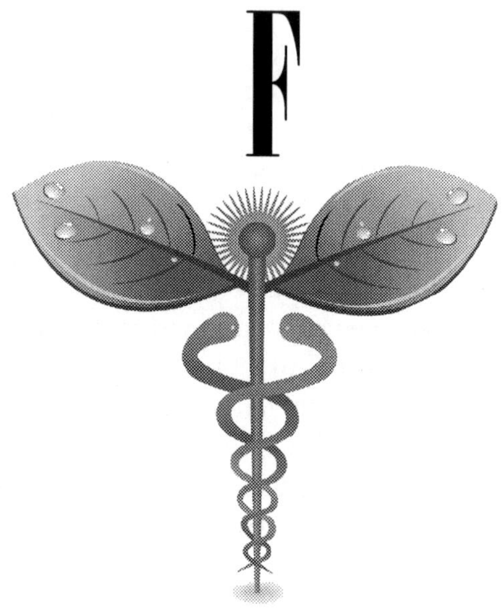

Fainting

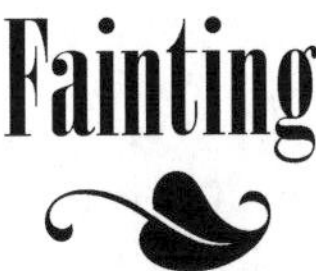

Passing Out / Blacking Out
Also see dizziness

Unlike what we often see or read in classic literature or modern movies, fainting is actually a much more complex process than many people believe. Heart palpitations, sweating and anxiety often accompany a brief, sudden loss of consciousness. People sometimes faint suddenly without any obvious reason. Unlike what we often see on screen, when people faint upon receiving disturbing news, in "real life" such episodes often accompany a combination of a sudden drop in blood pressure generated by strong emotion or anxiety, each in conjunction with low blood sugar.

Fainting Causes

Ultimately, in most instances a decreased blood flow to the brain causes the person to "pass out." This usually stems from either—or a combination of—specific factors including anemia, allergies, dehydration, nutritional deficiencies, and heart arrhythmias (slowing of pulse). This is an abnormal beating of the heart called "Bradycardia," low blood sugar, or insufficient levels of iron or magnesium. More serious conditions sometimes cause fainting such as mild strokes, (TIAs—Transient Ischemic Attacks). Benign or malignant tumors of the brain, and increased fluid pressure in the brain (hydro cephalus) must also be ruled out.

Additional Considerations

Gently revive someone who has fainted by using aromatherapy, using essential oils for rubbing under the nose—particularly black pepper, peppermint, rosemary, neroli, lavender or basil.

Fainting Treatments

Regulate blood pressure with herbs like olive leaf extract, Una de Gato known as "cat's claw," shepherds purse or unsweetened cocoa. Homeopaths sometimes recommend natural remedies such as Arsenicum album, Aconite and Ignatia. Practitioners of Ancient Chinese Medicine believe an ideal herb combination can improve bodily energy flow, stimulating blood pressure and circulation.

Always keep your body hydrated while also improving nutrition. Drink lots of filtered or spring water. Avoid processed meals, instead focusing on whole foods including vegetables and high-protein such as beans, bee pollen, chicken and fish. Eat moderate- or small-size meals throughout each day, accompanied by supplements containing magnesium, iron, Vitamin B and pantothetic acid.

Farsightedness & Nearsightedness

Hyperopia

Nearsighted people easily see objects close to them, while objects farther away seem blurry or completely out of focus. The opposite is true for farsighted people. Universally caused by corneal or eye muscle deficiencies, each affliction generates similar symptoms such as the inability to read for extended periods, eyestrain, headaches, blurred vision and a difficulty seeing or working up close.

Farsightedness and Nearsightedness Causes

In each condition, the retina fails to focus on visual images. Rather than focusing on the retina, the body attempts to focus either in front of or behind that vital tissue. This sometimes occurs when the cornea flattens or becomes shorter than normal. The vision problems occur because the tone within the ciliary muscle becomes insufficient, thereby unable to control lenses within one or both eyes.

Farsightedness and Nearsightedness Treatments

Various risks are associated with treatments offered by so-called traditional medicine for both farsightedness and nearsightedness. For farsightedness, standard medical practitioners usually recommend surgery or prescription lenses—eyeglasses or contact lenses.

Yet corrective lenses can cause a lack of depth perception, an increased reaction to artificial light, a worsening of the condition by decreasing the sensitivity of eye muscles, and inflamed corneas, a condition that doctors call "microbial keratitis."

Corrective surgeries for farsightedness and nearsightedness also pose potential complications. The most common procedures are PRK or photorefractive keratomy, and Lasik. Potential side effective are potentially catastrophic, such as optic nerve damage, the development of macular degeneration from holes in the macula, loss of detail, halos around lights, chronically dry eyes, and infections. The procedures also can detach or tear the retinas.

Alternative Remedies

Rather than risk problems from surgery or corrective lenses, some practitioners of natural medicine strive to train the eye muscles to focus. Such efforts are sometimes effective for both farsightedness and nearsightedness, partly because each condition result from macular problems. Yet any positive results happen gradually, rather than instantly as with lenses or surgeries.

Beneficial nutritional supplements can include vitamins A, C and E, and B-complex vitamins, plus zinc, zeaxthanin, beta-carotene, riboflavin, flavonoids, Selenium, taurine, riboflavin and N-acetyl-cysteine, sometimes called "NAC,." Lutein, Lycopene, and bilberry extract.

Homeopaths recommend diets rich in antioxidants and minerals. Typical foods here include carrots, purple berries, mangoes, and purple, red or orange bell peppers. Get additional help from parsley, celery, yellow squash, tomatoes and citrus fruits.

Also high on the list are red or purple grapes, melons, cherries, plums and purple berries.

Organic egg yolks prove beneficial thanks to high carotenoid content, while a mix of agave or raw honey with unsweetened cocoa also can help.

Fertility

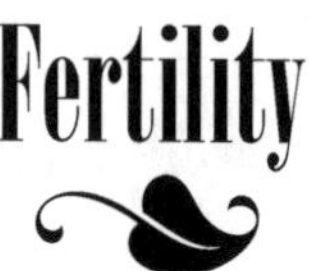

Sperm Count / Impotence

Also see Sexual Dysfunction

The instance of infertility problems in the U.S. culture is far more prevalent than many people believe, perhaps due to environmental factors—particularly toxins. By some accounts, about 4 million of the estimated 10 million such cases in the United States involve low sperm counts. The remaining 6 million instances involve female fertility problems. Although the problem is serious on a widespread scale, research indicates that half of these adults will eventually conceive, about half without seeking medical help.

Ultimately for many couples the much-wanted results occur by continually and regularly trying to conceive simply by "doing what comes naturally," a phrase inspired by the family-oriented hit Broadway musical "Annie Get Your Gun."

Infertility Causes

Besides physical damage caused by pesticides or environmental toxins like vehicle exhaust and industrial or household poisons, overly tight underwear is thought to sometimes contribute to low sperm counts. When worn too snuggly, such garments can create temperatures non-conducive to the healthful growth of sperm. Some researchers believe that men in cooler climates—particularly those avoiding tight underwear—produce more boys. Men living in cold climates apparently have more boys. Drugs and prostate issues also can impact sperm counts. Overall, men typically produce less sperm as they age. Women having polycystic ovaries (PCOS) have increased problems with fertility.

Other infertility problems sometimes occur for "obvious" reason. Namely, the man and woman fail to mate at an ovulation time of the month ideal for fertilization. Tobacco and alcohol worsens the problem in men. Further hampering chances for successful fertilization, some foods contain harmful toxins that lower fertility in both men and women. Common culprits here include nitrates, caffeine, sulfates, MSG, estrogen blockers and aromatase inhibitors.

Infertility Treatments

Couples experiencing infertility issues should have sex only when the woman ovulates. For many couples going for nearly one full month without orgasms or sexual release builds up overall hormones and sperm counts—while also accelerating sex drive.

Men should strive to ejaculate less frequently, allowing the density of ejaculate and sperm to build until entering women during ovulation. Guys who avoid alcohol while increasing their zinc intake boost their chances of successful fertilization.

Another key factor involves caring for the prostate, particularly by exercising regularly and also refraining from sitting for extended periods, or prolonged cycling.

Of course, women need to regularly track their menstrual cycles. Increase the chances of pregnancy by having intercourse just before or during ovulation.

Women can boost their reproductive system by drinking plenty of red raspberry leaf tea, before, during and after pregnancy. Maca root can increase fertility. Additional helpful herbs include ginseng, black cohosh and milk thistle.

Men and women should consider getting their livers, blood and colons cleansed while avoding environmental toxins.

Fibromyalgia

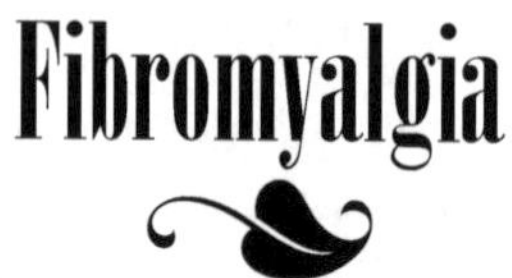

Also see Muccle Cramps, Viral Infections, Backache, Chronic Fatigue, Fibromyalgia

Some medical professionals mistakenly believe that physical inactivity can cause fibromyalgia, best described as muscle pain throughout the body. To the contrary, this condition that can cause muscles to weaken and atrophy typically occurs among physically active people.

Fibromyalgia occurs as "post-traumatic" due to physical trauma caused by injury or accidents, or in a "primary" form due to no specific or foreseeable cause.

Among common symptoms are insomnia, dizziness, headaches, irritability, increased sensitivities and allergies and mood swings. Other frequent symptoms include a heightened sensitivity to sounds, smells, cold and light, upper back pain, depression, anxiety, painful menstruation and a painful rib cage, upper back, knees or hips.

Fibromyalgia Causes

Chronic fatigue syndrome is sometimes blamed. (See that section.) Also, physicians usually blame sleep disorders, low serotonin levels, malfunctions in thalamus systems, poisoning from heavy metals and environmental toxins and hormone imbalances, particularly of the essential and natural human growth hormone. (HGH)

Fibromyalgia Treatments

Reduce pain and symptoms of fibromyalgia with nutritional supplements containing lipotrophic factors, zinc, magnesium, selenium, eicosapentaenoic acid commonly called "EPA," Vitamin C, Vitamin E and Vitamin B3.

Restore the body's natural muscle balance with bodywork

or exercise, improving nerve function and turning on joints that have been ravaged by the condition. Cleanse the body of wastes or toxins that can perpetuate or continue such conditions.

To treat the pain directly without addressing the underlying cause, try acupuncture targeting any bothersome muscles and muscles. Eliminating these pains can, in turn, fortify the body's natural ability to bring vital nutrients and oxygen to these bodily areas.

Eat foods easy on the digestive system and helpful in boosting immunity. Use more than your usual amounts of coconut oil or butter, flaxseed oil and virgin olive oil. Take small amounts of quinoa, beans and tofu, plus healthy amounts of organic free-range eggs, dark leafy greens and vegetables.

The many helpful herbs in eliminating, preventing or reducing fibromyalgia pain include raw, pure cocoa helpful in boosting the brain's serotonin levels, and fish oil supplements to reduce inflammation. Boost the immune system and reduce inflammation with tinctures taken three times daily of licorice, devil's claw, Echinacea, black cohosh, dandelion, olive leaf extract and cat's claw (una d'gato).

Push harmful toxins from the digestive system with Bentonite clay, and enhance digestion with cinnamon and cayenne. For additional pain relief, topically apply capsaicin cream, also reducing tension and anxiety with chamomile.

Fibrosis

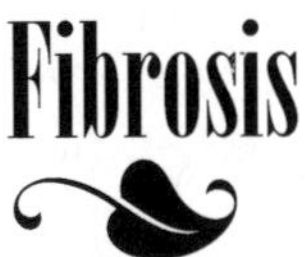

Also see Scarring, Cysts

Primarily suffered by people as they age, fibrocystic disease and the buildup of fiber-containing or fibrous tissue occurs when natural fibrin within the body is reduced by enzymes. An excessive buildup of fibrin, particularly in people as they get older, can reduce the size and function of vital organs.

The problem is so prevalent that at least half of women between ages 35 and 50 are prone to fibrocystic problems in their breasts. Scar tissue forms when connective tissue thickens within supporting tissues in the breasts. Some physicians blame an excessive estrogen buildup, while genetic components also apply. Typical symptoms include painful breasts during or before menstruation, and lumpy sections at the upper and outer perimeters of the breasts.

Fibrosis Causes

Researchers blame excessive estrogen, genetics, birth control pills and caffeine.

Fibrosis Treatments

Difficult to correct or cure, fibrosis is usually the target of efforts to slow its progression. Yet the condition sometimes disappears if treatments begin early, or with aging.

Hydrate the body the body by drinking lots of water, preferably carbon activated water to fortify the body's mineral retention. Containing salt and sugar makeup similar to blood plasma, coconut water also works well for hydration.

Increase Vitamin C while using low-dose rather than powerful birth control pills. Initially take daily 400 IU levels of Vitamin E to eliminate pain and resume comfort levels, and if those doses fail to raise blood pressure eventually increase those levels to 800 IU daily.

Meantime, take antioxidants, particularly pine bark extract, berries and pure cocoa. Along with the Vitamin C, also eat more bioflavonoid—particularly from citrus fruit, seahawthorn, and mangoes. Avoid caffeinated drinks if possible.

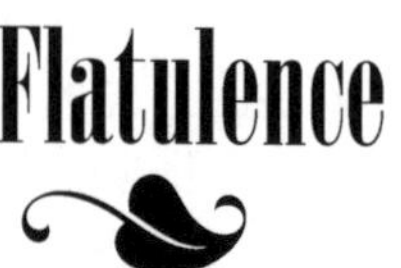

Flatulence

Gas, also see Digestion, Colon and Intestinal Health

Some people concoct wild stories to blame their pets after

hearty meals, although various effective natural strategies exist to correct this problem.

The trick here usually entails avoiding foods that cause excessive gas, particularly beans or high-oxygen and high-methane foods that contain substances upon which gas-producing bacteria like to eat. High-sulfur foods like milk, dairy products and eggs are common offenders, along with Brussels sprouts and cabbage.

The "trick" in preventing odiferous gas hinges on minimizing or preventing sulfur dioxide and nitrogen from a state of "volatile combustion."

Gas Causes

A health check-up is sometimes recommended or highly advisable, because chronic gas sometimes results from serious intestinal disorders, diabetes, poor liver function or thyroid imbalances, pancreatic enzyme problems, gluten allergies, and irritable bowel syndrome.

The so-called explosion of foul-smelling gasses generally ignites when gasses naturally produced within the digestive tract "ingested air," either swallowed or eaten. Ultimately, too much bad bacteria within the digestive tract generate intestinal gasses, usually the result of poor diets or specific foods.

For people lacking adequate levels of "good bacteria" in their guts, the "bad bacteria" takes over to ultimately generate the odiferous gasses.

This sometimes occurs after either unknowingly or haphazardly eaten foods or beverages that destroys good bacteria or creates bad bacteria.

Certain medications including antibiotics are sometimes to blame, while tap water loaded with fluoride or chlorine ravage or completely destroy good bacteria.

Excessive blood sugar sometimes serves as a breeding ground for bad bacteria, resulting in gas or constipation. Some of the worst foods are baking powder, risen breads, cheese, beer, wine, dried fruit and vinegar.

Gas Treatments

Try probiotics including acidophilus and bifidophilus beneficial in assisting "good bacteria." Meantime, you should avoid substances known to kill the helpful microorganisms. This means avoiding drugs and particularly antibiotics.

Use iodine to minimize or prevent bloating while, assisting normal thyroid function and relieving gas. Eat yogurts high in acidophilus, and also after meals enjoy non-yogurt natural foods like anise and fennel seeds. Carbon tablets can minimize acid indigestion that sometimes causes gas. For added benefit, enjoy kelp and before meals drink water containing a few drops of anise oil or peppermint.

G

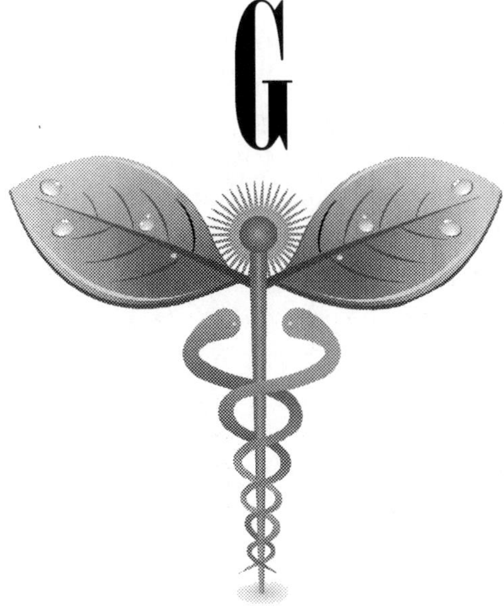

Glaucoma

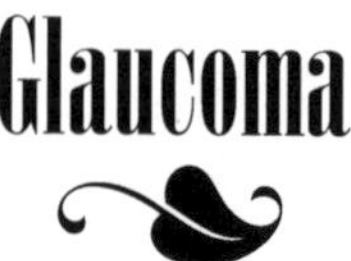

Also see Macular Degeneration, Cataracts

When fluid builds to abnormal levels, causing increased intraorbital pressure within the eyeball, glaucoma develops—the second leading cause of blindness in the United States behind cataracts. The fluid buildup destroys or damages the vital and necessary optic nerve and retina. Sadly, many people fail to realize that they suffer from glaucoma until it's "too late," past the point where irreversible damage has occurred.

First, peripheral vision fades, followed by the gradual onset of blindness. The vision loss is so gradual that many people fail to realize they suffer from this condition. Headaches, tunnel vision, vomiting and nausea are among common symptoms. Some individuals have difficulty seeing at night even when using eyewear, and the sensation of seeing halos around lights is a common complaint.

Most people suffering from glaucoma suffer from the "open-angle" variety, when the natural draining of fluid from the eye dissipates or fails altogether. In the other form, "closed-angle," the eyeball feels hard when touched due to a quick buildup of pressure caused by fluid.

Glaucoma Causes

Injuries, nutritional deficiencies, diabetes, genetics and premature aging are among causes. Children, teens and young adults can have glaucoma. Yet most instances seem to develop in step with the aging process. Diabetes, high blood pressure and allergies are sometimes blamed. Additional suspected causes are drugs known to change or regulate body fluids, everything from tetracycline and steroids to diuretics, antidepressants, blood pressure drugs and antihistamines.

Glaucoma Treatments

Some patients benefit from acupuncture or chelation alternative therapies. Take daily supplements containing taurine, riboflavin, vitamins A, C, E and E-complex, plus magnesium, lutein, lycopene, alpha-lipoic acid, and beta-carotene. When outdoors only use sunglasses having polarized lenses. Exercise the eyes to reduce facial pressure, particularly near those tissues. Avoid unnecessary eyestrain from using computers for extended periods or too much TV.

Avoid alcohol, caffeine, sugar, and all processed or fried foods. Instead, benefit from carotenoid-rich food, particularly organic egg yolks.

Benefit from foods rich in antioxidants such as citrus fruit, mangoes, melons, spinach, tomatoes, parsley, carrots, bell peppers, purple berries and dark-green leafy vegetables.

Gout

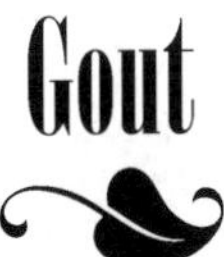

Also see Arthritis

An extremely painful disease, gout strikes when uric acid crystals build up in the joints. Three out of every four people with gout suffer extreme pain in the big toe. Yet many typical Americans apparently fail to realize that gout also can strike the spine, fingers, ankle, elbow, heel, instep, wrist or knee. Ninety percent of cases occur in men.

Gout Causes

Scientists admit they have failed to pinpoint an exact, universal cause for gout. Some researchers believe the vital organic purine compound within the body malfunctions, wreaking havoc on uric acid levels within the body. Some people with gout have an increase in uric acid production, too much of the substance and even a combination of these conditions. A rapid breakdown of tumors from chemotherapy also can cause gout. Heredity plays a big role in this disease.

The worst pain impacts tissues near or around the joint, or when patients try to move areas where crystals have accumulated. Some patients complain of low-grade fever. Joint stiffness and severe pain is often accompanied by warmness, redness or swelling.

Gout Treatments

Take 50 milligrams of niacin and 3 grams of Vitamin C with each meal. Make tea using bilberry, an effective natural arthritis treatment. The natural diuretic sarsaparilla, or burdock root can be helpful. Bilberry helps stabilize collagen. Take xanthine oxidase to counteract an enzyme that promotes the body's production of uric acid. Reduce swelling with burdock root, and benefit from bromelain found in pineapples.

For many years people in England have used natural beverages and substances to effectively control or to eliminate gout. After consuming water and honey to minimize the potentially raspy taste, horsetail herbs, apple cider vinegar and black cherry juice are formidable natural remedies.

A continual healthful diet low in purine can help by robbing or lessening any opportunity for the body to process that substance into harmful uric acid. Some foods and beverages help neutralize purine, particularly distilled water, diluted celery juice, fresh fruits and vegetables. Cherries and strawberries can be particularly powerful. The many high-purine foods to avoid include sugar, yeast, meat, fish, white flour, cauliflower, chocolate, lentils, asparagus, peas, spinach and mushrooms.

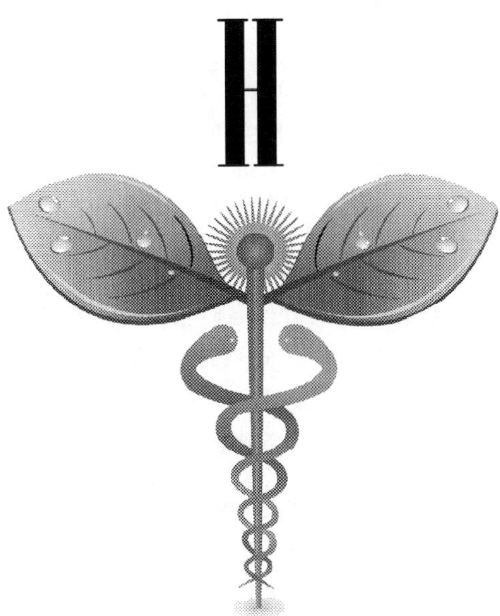
II

Hair (Graying)

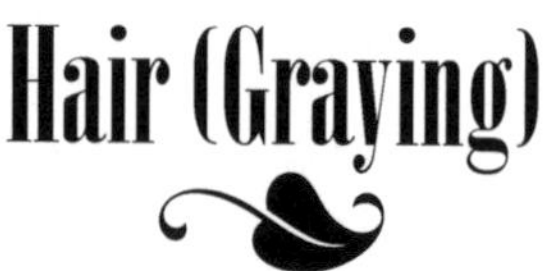

Also see Hair Loss

Some people go prematurely gray while others retain youthful hair well into their advanced years. The quick but unnatural remedy involves dying the hair. Yet natural treatments for addressing the underlying causes exist as well.

In specific instances, homeopaths occasionally suspect decreased or insufficient functioning of the pancreas, kidneys or spleen, conditions triggered by stress. Using natural remedies can help the person feel younger while also returning youthful colors.

Gray Hair Causes

Most instances come from the body's natural decreases in estrogen and testosterone as we age. Excess caffeine or stress can force the body to produce too much cortisol, reducing the levels of natural hormones that once produced youthful-looking hair.

Gray Hair Treatments

Strive to reduce stress that generates cortisol, a substance which robs hair of its healthy, colorful appearance. While avoiding harsh chemicals that color the hair, take B-complex vitamins to boost natural hormone levels. Benefit from increased circulation derived from pure cocoa, green tea extract, and cat's claw. Build estrogen and testosterone with supplements rich in DHEA, technically called "dehydroepiandrosterone," and also ginseng, and biotin. Genetics plays a major role.

Hair Loss

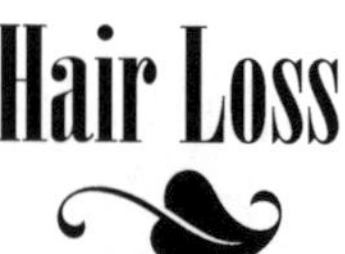

Male Pattern Baldness / Alopecia / Female Hair Loss

Also see Hair (Graying)

Most hair loss strikes men due to genetic factors impacting

certain individuals of their gender. Yet many people fail to realize that certain natural remedies can significantly slow the loss of hair. For men natural remedies can reduce hair thinness to levels experienced up to 10 years earlier. Such treatments typically fail to reverse hair loss in all instances, but some men report such benefits.

Hair Loss Causes

Inadequate nutrition is sometimes cited, a condition sometimes reversed by adding more minerals, vitamins and protein to the diet.

Poor circulation sometimes prevents nutrients necessary for growing healthy hair from reaching the scalp.

Stress adversely impacts hormones, stopping or curtailing hair production. Most hair loss stems from genetic factors inherited from a maternal grandparent, impacting both men and women. Hormonal imbalances also are blamed, particularly when the body produces too much of the androgen male hormone. This factor sometimes causes women to lose hair following childbirth or menopause, due to excess androgen levels coupled with decreases in estrogen. In cancer patients, both chemotherapy and radiation therapy to the scalp are the main culprits.

Hair Loss Treatments

Exercise to reduce stress and to improve blood circulation, which also can be improved with the natural cat's claw or "Una de Gato" substance from the Amazon.

Topical applications, herbs, exercise and massage can stimulate the scalp. Changes in lifestyle habits and herbs can significantly help hair grow but not in all cases. Scientists say more study is needed to prove or disprove the effectiveness of such natural treatments.

Additional hair loss is sometimes prevented with fruit, grains nuts and beans, all with high inositol content. High-fat and high-protein diets are often blamed, so men and women experiencing hair loss should cut down on such foods. Eat more vegetables and fruit, while reducing starches and protein. Take more Vitamin E, while also mixing alpha-lipoic acid, the horsetail herb, and organic silica with biotin.

Many treatments strive to increase blood flow to the scalp. Acupuncture reportedly offers apparent benefits. Some practitioners of natural medicine urge patients to stop smoking, which damages DNA—prohibiting or restricting hair growth. Researchers identify alcohol as another culprit.

Try to prevent complete hair loss with the oatstraw and horsetail herbs. Practitioners of Eastern medicine believe that castor oil and red sage help regenerate hair growth.

Hangover

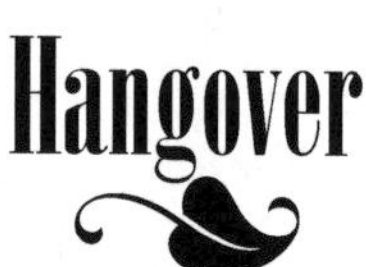

Needless to say, hangovers notoriously cause some people to regret drinking alcohol. Many individuals fail to realize that hangovers sometimes are far worse than merely a “bad headache.” The condition can lead to infection, weaked immunity and thereby increased vulnerability to disease. Just as destructive, hangovers can damage liver functions, and inflame the digestive system.

Hangover Causes

Excess alcohol consumption pushes toxic chemicals into the kidneys and liver, while dehydrating the body and seriously lowering blood sugar. Regular excess alcohol drinking exacerbates the problem with premature aging, weight gain, diabetes, and serious damage to the stomach, liver, esophagus and bladder.

Hangover Treatments

To push alcohol and toxins from their bodies, some people try hot showers or hot steam baths.

The best way to treat or prevent hangover is to avoid drinking alcohol or at the very least to minimize such consumption. Drink ample amounts of pure water between alcoholic drinks, and also right before bedtime and right after awakening. Improve the effectiveness of water by adding a teaspoon of sugar and a pinch of salt to a large glass. Amid a hangover, re-hydrate the body with lime juice, sugar and cayenne pepper added to tomato juice. If you feel a need to drink alcohol, eat lots of food beforehand.

Drink diuretic herbs to support or to help protect the kidneys. Bitter herbs can help minimize the adverse side affects, particularly dandelion root, mugwort, and gentian.

Headaches

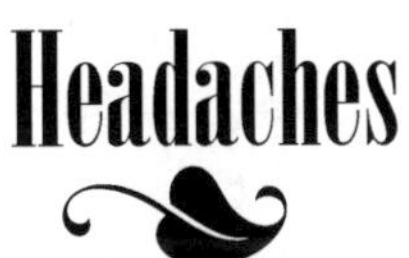

Migraine Headaches
Also see Stress, Allergies, Congestion

Most of us suffer headaches at some point in our lives, an unwanted symptom so prevalent that a mast majority of people in the Western Hemisphere have complained of this problem.

The natural substance of aspirin and other low-dose less natural substances are often used. Practitioners of natural medicines list lots of additional preventions and treatments.

Severe migraine headaches are usually unilateral and may generate localized vision loss and nausea after the head suffers a slow, gradually building throb. Some migraines stretch for days, actually starting with the vision problems and nausea.

Headache Causes

The wide variety of known causes range from premenstrual headaches associated with hormonal imbalances, sinus congestion, stress, eye strain, environmental toxins and allergies. (Each of these symptoms has natural remedies, as listed in this guide.)

Additional Considerations

Relax tense muscles by massaging both sides of the head under the two ridges, releasing nerve pressure that sometimes leads to migraines or common headaches. Non-traditional acupuncture sometimes works. Persistent headaches demand medical attention and this could signal a benign or malignant brain tumor.

Headache Treatments

Dehydration that can occur in any season can generate headaches, so try to relieve pain by drinking a few full glasses of water—a strategy that gives some people almost immediate pain relief.

People who suffer migraines should pay close attention to what they eat. Some researchers blame food allergies for causing nine out of every 10 migraines. Chocolate, caffeine, preservatives and colorings are often suspected. Chronic migraine suffers should gradually eliminate specific foods from their diets in efforts to pinpoint apparent causes.

The most common culprits are shell fish, peanut butter, peanuts, coffee, soda, and dairy or cheese products. High fructose corn syrup, sugar, wheat, gluten, MSG, sulfites, vinegar, pickled products and preservatives generate equal concern.

Everyone should be wary of non-aspirin over-the-counter pain relievers, and even powerful pain-relieving pharmaceuticals, because those substances weaken immunity, and injure the stomach, liver or kidneys. Prolonged use of non-aspirin pain relievers weakens health. For best results, try taking the substance that original versions of aspirin were made from, white willow bark extract.

To reduce stress, try massaging the head with lavender, used as a remedy for thousands of years. Other natural remedies to soothe the vascular system while controlling blood pressure include mint extract, wild yam, pure cocoa, valerian root, olive leaf extract, turmeric, chamomile, skullcap, passion fruit extract and bay leaves.

Heart Disease

Also see Cholesterol, Anti-Inflammatory, Blood Pressure, Cardiovascular Health

Many types of heart ailments generate severe danger or health problems. Obesity, cholesterol and arterial plaque comprise just a handful of the many causes or symptoms. In fact, many people fail to realize that the causes are far more extensive than the additional potential factors of atherosclerosis, cholesterol and high blood pressure. Within developed countries, heart disease kills more people than any other disease or affliction.

Heart Disease Causes

Contrary to popular belief, the main culprit in heart attacks is something other than cholesterol. Most people who suffer such life threatening conditions have normal cholesterol levels. Just as disturbing, according to some reports, most people with high cholesterol never suffer heart attacks.

An estimated 13 million Americans take cholesterol-lowering drugs called "statins" that endangers the liver and cause muscle aches.

Even so, inflammation is a significant factor in heart disease, not just cholesterol. Foods or habits leading to inflammation include a sedentary lifestyle, advancing age, diabetes, insufficient nutrients, high blood pressure, smoking and toxins.

Heart Disease Prevention and Treatments

Scientists and homeopaths have identified various specific methods and strategies for attacking and preventing various heart conditions. Among them:

Fortify: Strengthen heart muscles with 20 milligrams of potassium and 100 milligrams of Q10, also called Co-Q10.

Prevention: Studies indicate that the levels of DHEA or

dehydroepiandrosterone lower with age, linked to heart disease, arthritis, diabetes and obesity. Some researchers believe that taking just 10 milligrams of DHEA daily can reduce heart disease deaths by nearly half.

Inflammation: Use anti-inflammatory herbs and foods. Regularly enjoy the most effective herbs, primarily Vitamin C, milk thistle, cat's claw, black cohlosh, garlic, motherwort, wild yam, white willow and pine bark extract.

Flabby hearts (Cardiomyopathy) : Homeopaths believe that selenium improves this condition. Human growth hormone is often beneficial.

Heart palpitations: To calm the heart, blood pressure and nervous system, use spearmint, Saint John's wort, leonuri, eucalyptus, valerian root and hawthorne berry. All have hypotensive antispasmodic qualities.

Arterial plaque: Address or prevent this condition, along with arterial and coronary inflammation with a consistent enzyme regimen containing red algae, primrose oil, EFA's, colloidal silver, red Chinese yeast, Co-Q-10, aged garlic and Vitamin E.

Clogging arteries: Although strengthening blood vessel walls, whenever Vitamin C is not present the lipoprotein-a within arterial plaque also clogs the same vessels. So, take daily doses of the vital natural nutrient to fight the arterial plaque. At least twice daily added to meals, cut homocysteine levels with: TMG or trimethlglycine, 500 to 1,000 milligrams; Vitamin B12 or methylcobalamine, 1 milligram; and folic acid, 800 mcg; and Vitamin B6, 100 mgm.

Heart Palpatations

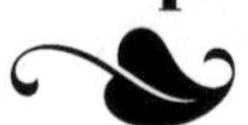

Arrhythmia / Ectopia, also see Thyroid Imbalance, Adrenal Imbalance, Anxiety, Hypoglycemia

The romanticism often featured in movies or novels of

skipping heart beats can actually occur. For countless generations doctors have known that suddenly seeing an inspiring object, panic, feeling love, shock and other strong emotions can intensify heartbeats. Usually such heart-skipping should cause little or no reason for worry, unless such conditions continue unabated at frequent intervals or cause fibrillation or flutter.

Such conditions could be a sign of abnormal heart functioning. So, remain watchful for unusual signs, such as lightheadedness, chest pains before or during palpitations. Visit a cardiologist if your heart races frequently for minutes or hours.

Heart Palpitation Causes

A healthy heart depends on reliable, steady and non-stop electrical impulses at a regular and healthful rate. Various bodily problems can cause this vital energy system to go haywire, essentially firing irregularities—thereby producing excessively heavy pounding or irregular and potentially dangerous rhythms. Some people suffer heart palpitations after exerting themselves too much, in some instances generating excess adrenaline or disrupting the healthful levels and rates of processing oxygen.

Panic attacks or extreme anxiety sometimes ignite the problem. Excessive medication, Grave's Disease and overactive thyroids are sometimes to blame. Too much caffeine sometimes sparks the problem. Sudden or excessive emotion can trigger these dangerous conditions. Fear, shock and panic sometimes force adrenaline to rush into overdrive. Severe coronary disease can trigger this condition.

Heart Palpitation Treatments

If suffering this condition, ask your medical professional to check for Grave's Disease or other thyroid imbalances. When hot flashes are involved, grapes can help slow the heart rate.

Take plenty of vitamins B and C and E vitamins when stress, trauma or shock are the cause. For all forms of palpitations, cut all stimulants including caffeine from your diet. Reduce blood pressure with fish, fruit and vegetables. Potassium and magnesium also help, derived from supplements or natural foods like nectarines and bananas. Supplements also should include helpful amounts of magnesium, which helps relax the lungs, chest and heart. Some of the most effective natural foods and herbs include chamomile, motherwort, mint, Chinese skullcap and hawthorn berries.

Heartburn

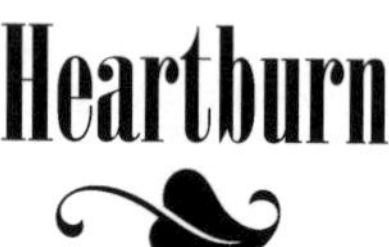

Gastroesophageal Reflux Disease (GERD), Acid Indigestion
Also see Digestion

Some people fail to realize that the heart actually has nothing to do with the bothersome and uncomfortable condition that we call "heartburn." Rather than occurring in this vital organ, the discomfort or acute pain actually occurs near that area. Heartburn commonly in the lower esophagus.

The condition can last for days in some people, and pain levels vary. In all instances, never take antacids sold over the counter. Contrary to popular believe, some heartburn actually results from insufficient levels of stomach acids—not too much of it.

Besides striving to reduce acid when more is needed, when used long-term the sodium bicarbonate and aluminum from antacids can cause alkalosis.

Heartburn Prevention and Treatment

Restore the stomach's normal balance of acidity and alkalinity, a level commonly known as "pH." Stop heartburn while aiding indigestion with a teaspoon of apple cider vinegar high in acetic acid—which helps digestion.

To cut down on gas, acid and heartburn, take carbon tablets and also drink a glass of warm water containing a teaspoon of baking soda—but not harmful, dangerous aluminum-rich baking powder.

Never overeat, because the buildup of pressure in a filled stomach can push food up toward the esophagus. Get quick relief from any acid burning sensation by drinking cold milk to line the stomach and esophagus.

Avoiding certain foods serves as the easiest and safest method for prevention and treatment and prevention. So, never eat or at least cut down on foods that rob the stomach of acids, particularly caffeine, tomato sauces, and spicy or fried foods. Among other prevention tips:

Smoking: Avoid smoking tobacco, especially before meals.

Healthful bacteria: Fortify or increase "good bacteria" in the stomach and digestive tract by taking probiotic or enzymes daily

Unhealthful combinations: Never simultaneously drink wine and caffeine, and never mix fresh salads or fruit with other foods. Refrain from unnecessarily adding sugar to food. Wait for awhile after a meal to have dessert.

Chewing: Rather than quickly swallowing, chew your food well. This maximizes the efficiency of enzymes in breaking down food.

Moderation: Never overeat, thereby preventing pressure buildups that cause heartburn.

Alcohol: Drink a maximum of one wine or beer nightly.

Avoid: Never eat or at least cut down on: pasta, refined white sugar, or white bread made with refined carbohydrates; highly caffeinated tea, coffee and chocolate; tomato sauce; and fried foods.

Hemorrhoids

Also see Constipation, Colon and Intestinal Health

Common among people older than 49, irritating and painful hemorrhoids sometimes cause bowel movement difficulty or constipation that hampers or prolongs healing. Swollen or painful tissues sometimes hamper life so much that one out of every eight Americans ages 50 and older seeks surgical treatment.

Mild cases outside the body cause anal-area irritation, discomfort or itching. Some hemorrhoids develop inside the rectum, creating lesions that lead to bloody stools.

Hemorrhoid Causes

Rectal cancer is suspected among seniors who suddenly get hemorrhoids. Some women suffer hemorrhoids after childbirth due to strain that causes inflamed or swollen veins. For most hemorrhoid sufferers, constipation, sedentary lifestyles, improper diets that lead to straining to pass stools or failing to drink enough water are among common causes or contributing factors.

Hemorrhoid Treatments

Avoid alcohol, hot spices and dairy products, especially cheeses. Use natural balms, particularly witch hazel extract found in most drugstores, for immediate pain relief. Many over-the-counter hemorrhoid treatments contain this ingredient. Using a cotton ball to apply the extract or aloe vera gel directly onto hemorrhoids is a much less expensive alternative.

To soften stools, along with Vitamin C, drink lots of water and eat raw vegetables. Pure olive oil and coffee also can help. Boost healing by adding chlorophyll to your diet, prevalent in barley, wheatgrass, Spirulina, Chlorella and alfalfa. Quinine bark serves as another good natural treatment.

Hepatitis

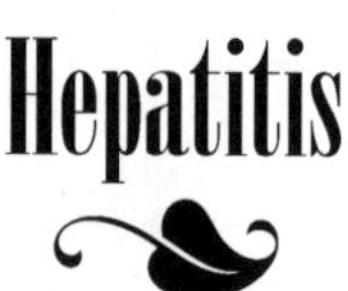

Also see Liver and Gallbladder Health

Many patients have yellowish eyes and skin, suffering discolored dark urine, vomiting, nausea, stomach pain, fatigue, and joint pain when suffering from active acute hepatitis—a potentially life threatening condition which may destroy the liver.

Hepatitis Causes

Viral infections generate most cases of Hepatitis A, B and C. Toxins from food, pharmaceuticals, alcohol and drug abuse are among other possible causes. Found in human stools, hepatitis A is a contagious and potentially dangerous condition. The blood-borne varieties of Hepatitis B, C and D are contracted in direct person-to-person contact through needles and blood transfusions.

Additional Considerations

Analgesic products like Tylenol contain acetaminophen, which endangers people suffering from hepatitis.

Hepatitis Treatments

Use microscopic particles of high-quality colloidal silver as a powerful anti-viral. Strengthen the immune system to fight hepatitis virus via Vitamin C administered via IV. Benefit from high-quality colloidal silver, a powerful anti-viral. Take glutathione, sometimes called "glutamine," to strengthen the liver, also using milk thistle consistently over to cleanse the organ. Add selenium and alpha lipoic acid to heal the liver.

Practitioners of Chinese Medicine also clean the organ using "liver tea," comprised of licorice, auratium fruit, bupleurum, white peony, citrus peel, ligusticum and cyperus. Without food, drink at least two 12-ounce glasses of daily after boiling the brew and steeping for at least two hours. (This also dissolves kidney stones and gallstones when taken over a two-week period.)

Burdock tea, another remedy often used in Traditional Chinese Medicine, helps clean the blood while boosting liver function. For each cup of water add 12 teaspoons of dried burdock root powder. Herbal Quercetin has been effective in hepatitis.

Herniated Disc

Under healthful conditions, the vertebrae are protected or cushioned by spinal discs. But bulges comprised of the soft inner core sometimes erupt when a disc's outer shell weakens.

Extreme pain occurs when these bulges or herniated discs press along any of the spine's many nerves. (This should not be confused with "ruptured discs," a completely different condition. Unlike herniated discs, a ruptured disc is completely debilitating. Ruptured discs require X-rays or imaging tests to diagnose, and usually surgery to repair.

Herniated discs can lead to potentially excruciating health problems such as incontinence, malfunctioning bowel control, numbness, weakness and especially pain. These factors or conditions can in turn lead to disturbing or serious symptoms in the limbs, weakness, tingling or numbness.

Herniated Disc Causes

Besides weak bones, genetic factors and advancing age, common causes or contributing factors include inflexibility, weak muscles, placing the body in unusual positions, heavy lifting, falls, motor vehicle accidents, and osteoporosis.

Herniated Disc Treatments

The "best treatment" for herniated discs starts with prevention. Remain extremely careful if you must lift heavy objects. Some health experts recommend keeping the back straight at all times, even when standing or walking. Exercise, stay in shape, get lots of sunshine and use relaxation techniques like yoga. Avoid dairy, acidic food, coffee and fluoride.

Improve overall results by intermixing rest and exercise. Also, subject the affected area with warm baths or direct heat from pads, sunshine or sun lamps.

Some doctors recommend surgery. But before doing so try non-traditional accupuncture treatments, which reportedly may have far greater results than operations.

Also, without initially going completely upside down, use an inversion swing. Start slowly, first going only partly upside down.

Herbs can help with digestive enzymes, particularly rose hips, nettle leaf, prickly ash bark, and marshmallow root. For additional help, try chondroitin, hyaluronic acid, MSM, glucosamine and collagen. Numerous medical facilities report excellent results using magnetic therapy targeting these hernias. Some practitioners of natural medicine claim that magnetic beds and magnets relieve pain when applied to the affected area.

Far infrared matts provide a healthing quality and relieve pain.

Herpes

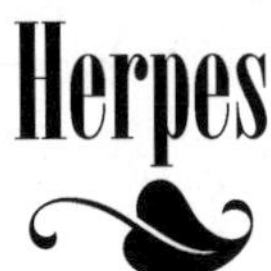

HSV / Cold Sore / Fever Blister / HHV-6

Herpes spreads from person-to-person, a virus that doctors list as "epidemic" or "easily transferable." There are numerous types of herpes, most described as "unsightly" or uncomfortable at the very least. Specific areas of the body are affected, and differing symptoms occur, depending on the type of herpes or the method of transfer.

Genital herpes or herpes simplex ii are among the most widely known forms. As its name implies, the genital variety occurs in the genital region. Avoid this type by refraining from putting or allowing your genetalia to come into direct contact with the genitals of another person's body—particularly while the virus is "active."

Scabs form during pelvic area outbreaks, often accompanied by burning or fever following initial outbreaks. Genital herpes is particularly contagious during outbreaks. Seemingly random shedding phases occur, and the virus can spread at any time—even while the person thinks that he or she is in a "safe period."

Herpes simplex also occurs when coming into direct contact with another person's affected area, a contagious condition affecting the mouth or genitals. Blisters form, and the condition is particularly contagious during unpredictable outbreaks. At times women with herpes simplex lack any symptoms of the condition.

Long-term fatigue occurs during another lesser-known form of herpes, Epstein Barr Virus, which also causes mononucleosis. Also, chronic fatigues syndrome has been associated with the little-known Type 6 herpes (HHV-6), which has been reported to be present within the bodies of an estimated 6.65 billion people; these individuals have developed antibodies almost always effectively fighting the virus.

However, sometimes many years or even decades after initially coming into contact with Type 6 herpes, toxins, stress or weakened hormonal imbalances cause this virus to reactivate in adults.

Herpes Treatment and Prevention

Lead by the worst offender, stress, the most prevalent factors in generating herpes outbreaks are: malic acid, derived from concentrated fruit juice; sunburn; and the arginine amino acid from fruit juices, particularly orange juice.

Homeopaths administer or recommend numerous natural, harmless herpes remedies. Among the most powerful:

Zinc: In supplement form, this helps stop the spread within the body of herpes simplex, but not necessarily genital herpes. Overnight beneficial results sometimes occur by taking zinc and L-lysine, also chewing folic acid tablets. Zinc lowers the strength of herpes.

Neem: Good for treating oral and genital herpes, this should only be used by people who first carefully study its attributes, which to some people has an objectionable taste and smell, also likely to cause stains.

Garlic: Some research indicates that garlic effectively treats herpes simplex and genital herpes, although this herb is more famous for eradicating fungal infections.

L-Lysine: The herpes virus dies after eating the herb lorea, which contains the natural amino acid lysine that the virus mistakes for arginine. Important: People with liver conditions should never take lorea. Every morning and evening while taking lorea, be sure to avoid carbohydrates from bread and sugar, and also eat plenty of lean protein. Please note that too much arginine can block L-lysine from doing killing the virus. So eat plenty of foods high in L-lysine like grains, nuts and chocolate.

Balm: Topically apply Aloe Vera and lemon balm on herpes sores.

Licorice: Although considered a treat, this is actually a powerful pain reliever as formidable as steroids but without the serious medical complications. Either ingest as a tea or apply topically via a soaked bandage to the ulcer.

Vitamin C: This substantial antiviral and antioxidant can lower the occurrence of outbreaks, while boosting the immune system.

Sarsaparilla: Control outbreaks by taking sarsaparilla as a tea, also helpful in preventing the body from developing herpes if exposed.

Hiccups

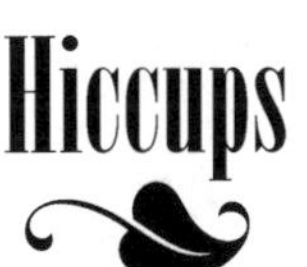

Rather than merely a amusing phenomena, hiccups can become serious when they persist. Long-term suffers of extended periods can suffer extreme fatigue or exhaustion.

Otherwise, in the vast majority of instances hiccups are harmless, usually disappearing within several minutes.

Hiccups Causes

The vocal chords suddenly close, when the diaphragm quickly contracts or due to an obstruction. Researchers usually blame too improper breathing or excess oxygen, conditions that can cause the diaphragm to suddenly contract. Malignant tumors involving the diaphragm can cause persistent hiccups.

Hiccup Treatments

The most common and usually ineffective methods for stopping hiccups range from drinking water while upside down to holding out the tongue until they disappear. Numerous natural techniques usually help (get a chest X-ray of symptoms persist.):

Drink: Amid an attack, take one part of castor oil with one part honey.

Aroma: The aroma of certain natural substances can help, particularly rosemary, pine, sesame, peppermint and anis. Breathe in the aromas of an otherwise dry cloth on which a few drops of the oils have been applied.

Breathing: Take a long, deep breath to maximum capacity before holding the air in your lungs for as long as possible. Exhale after a while before repeating the process at least two more times.

Alternative: Various non-traditional medicines or treatments can help, including hypnosis, massage, and acupressure.

Hives

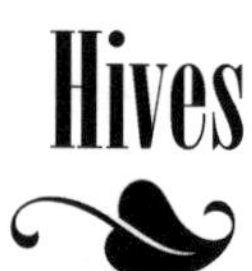

Dermographia / Heat Rash / Urticaria / Whales
Also see Allergies

White blotches surrounded by red patches on the skin mark the appearance of hives, raised bumps on the skin surface. Sometimes looking similar to insect bites or welts, hives appear in a variety of forms generated by various causes.

Although occasionally on the feet, hives usually erupt or form on the upper body, including the hands, arms, chest and back. Symptoms can last from a few minutes, to several hours or even days.

Doctors call hives "urticaria," named for a stinging nettle plant that can generate redness, skin rashes and itching.

Hives Causes

The body creates urticaria or hives as a defensive action against various conditions or allergies. Emotion is often a contributing factor, particularly depression or stress—sometimes exacerbating hives initially caused by other factors.

A wide range of allergies can cause hives, with offenders including dairy and meat. Some hive sufferers blame nuts, shellfish, citrus or tropical fruit, and strawberries. Such rashes also can be caused by exposure to natural or manmade atmospheric conditions like hot water, humidity and hot air.

Tight-fitting clothes can generate urticaria, particularly around the waistline from belts or on the chest or back from poorly fitted bras. The condition usually subsides within one hour, but can last several hours when reactions become intense.

Hives Treatments

Doctors have no "known universal cure" good for all instances of hives. Refrain from scratching red areas or hives, which worsens the condition.

Antihistamines (Benadryl) sold over-the-counter can relieve or eliminate symptoms. Yet for some the highest dosages available via such purchases of 10 milligrams are not enough.

People needing higher doses for treating hives usually require at least 25 milligrams. Remember, as stated elsewhere in this guide, antihistamines taken regularly over extended periods can rarely damage the kidneys and liver, and cause prostate swelling.

Adding to the challenge, antihistamine is an unnatural manufactured substance, and no known natural substances have its attributes. Even so, homeopaths have developed or identified natural remedies effective in minimizing the frequency or doses of antihistamine. Among the best:

Peppermint: Take in oil form, or drink as a tea.

Arnica cream: Applied topically to ease itching and redness.
Supplements: Vitamin B, Vitamin C and bromelain.
Herbs: Apis mel and Urtica Urens
Action: Reduce symptoms with body brushing and cold baths.

Human Papilloma Virus

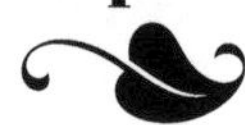

HPV / Cervical Cancer / Genital Warts / Plantar Warts / Vaginal Warts, also see Infection (Virus)

Commonly called HPV, the human papilloma virus has become an urgent topic throughout the media in recent years. A much-despised and unwanted verifiable cause of head and neck, anal, and cervical cancer in women, HPV is a sexually transmitted infection. In the United States an estimated 20 million people have HPV, many of them sexually active young adults.

For good reason, some worry and overall public concern stems from the disturbing fact that HPV can go undetected for years without symptoms. Such asymptomatic conditions generate a threat, an indisputable reason for women to get Pap smears.

Contrary to what advertisements might say, vaccinations fail to prevent or to cure HPV. Unscrupulous pharmaceutical companies try to scare the public into buying ineffective HPV vaccines, chemicals that can generate dangerous side effects.

HPV Causes

Any rumors are untrue about contracting HPV from toilet seats. Instead, the virus is transmitted via direct human-to-human contact. Almost any sexual contact can transfer the virus to another person, not just intercourse.

Treatments

HPV fails to pose any danger in a vast majority of cases. Early treatment can help obliterate threats or the seriousness of the virus.

Failing to take action early can prove fatal or life-threatening. Thus, medical checkups are necessary or highly advisable, particularly among women who might face the risk of cervical cancer.

Numerous topically applied natural remedies can effectively treat the virus, which affects the skin. These helpful remedies to applied daily for several weeks are liquid silver, Echinacea extract, Saint John's wort in liquid extract form, the best and most expensive tea tree oils and Artemesia.

Homeopaths insist that these work just as effectively as expensive medications prescribed by standard allopathic physicians.

Practitioners of natural medicine recommend oral supplements for use in conjunction with the topical remedies. These include as antioxidants flaxseed oil, green tea extract, pure cocoa, and pine bark extract. Boost the immune system with health-forming, nutrient rich foods and olive leaf extract. Additional antiviral protection can come orally from skullcap herbs, Echinacea and Saint John's wort.

Remove excess sugar, too much alcohol and processed foods from your diet, and also stop smoking.

Additional Considerations

HPV is transmitted via contact to any area of exposed skin, so condoms fail to provide complete protection against the virus. HPV infections have been linked to anal-genital and head-and-neck cancers as well.

Despite modern medical advances, doctors still lack a reliable method for detecting HPV in men. Although such examinations are not 100-percent reliable, men require visual inspections of their groin area because the most common signal in males comes from genital warts. For most guys who contract HPV the condition affecting only the skin disappears naturally without treatment and without generating severe health problems.

Any burning sensation a man might feel while urinating is

from something other than HPV, probably a bacterial infection effectively treated with oregano extract or garlic extract. Guys can control or avoid bacterial infections by striving to keep their body more alkaline than acidic, eating spinach, devil's claw, Echinacea, kale, green foods and Spirulina.

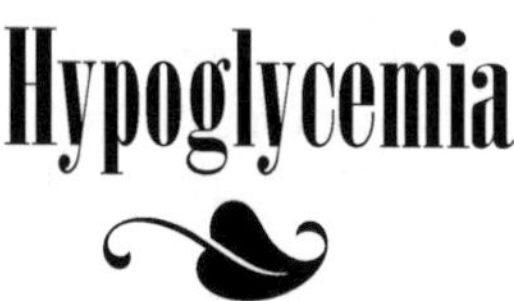

Hypoglycemia

Low Blood Sugar

Also see Candida, Adrenal Imbalance, Blood Pressure (Low)

People suffering hypoglycemia can suffer a general lack of energy and "the shakes," or disturbed mental conditions such as forgetfulness and fear when blood sugars dip. Emotional outbursts and mental imbalances sometimes coupled with confusion can make a person feel "as if I'm losing my mind."

Symptoms can become so disturbing that some patients experience heart palpitations, or insomnia that generates a continual desire to lie down. A sudden desire for food, particularly sweets to boost blood sugar, and blurry vision can prove just as debilitating. Some patients occasionally feel okay before adverse symptoms resume.

Hypoglycemia Causes

Scientists have identified two types of hypoglycemia:

Reactive hypoglycemia: Often a precursor to Type 2 diabetes, blood sugar goes extremely high before plummeting. This generates negative symptoms like fainting or dizziness due to a rapid change in blood sugar levels. Sweating, muscle cramps and nausea prove just as disturbing.

Conditioned hypoglycemia: The pancreas creates too much insulin after the person eats high-starch food or refined sugar. The person becomes extremely tired while the accelerated insulin production robs the body of healthful stable blood sugars.

Hypoglycemia Treatments

Many people suffering from either form of hypoglycemia are delighted upon discovering effective natural treatments and preventions exist—particularly if these remedies begin before the onset of Type 2 diabetes.

Avoid caffeine, refined starches, white sugar, fruit and alcohol. At least 20 minutes before breakfast, start each day by drinking two 12-ounce glasses of purified water. Avoid carbohydrates and sugar, making the day's first meal a fist-size portion of protein—thereby lessening or eliminating any desire for sweets.

Candida symptoms can mimic hypoglycemia, so some people mistakenly believe they have low blood sugar problems. (See the Candida section.) Daily for six weeks, each morning, take 1,000 milligrams of Vitamin C with 50 milligrams of pantothenic acid and 150 milligrams of adrenal cortex extract. Just before bed each night, take an additional 1,000 milligrams of Vitamin C and 500 milligrams of pantothenic acid.

The lightheadedness you once experienced when suddenly standing should disappear after this six-week regimen, while concentration improves and mental symptoms subside. Also, stabilize blood sugar with 200 micrograms of chromium picolinate added to food.

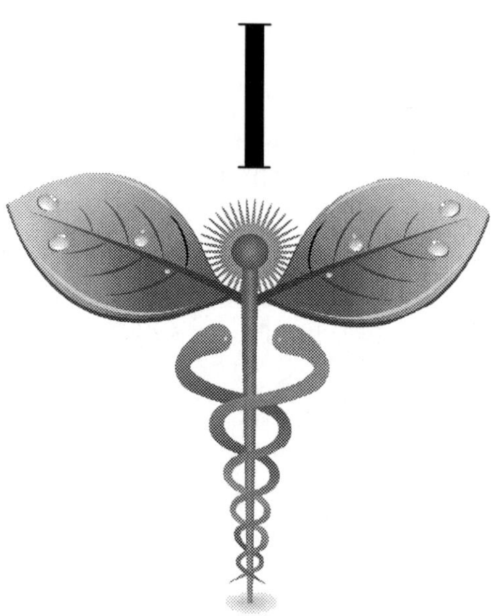
I

Immune System Health

Recovery from Illness / Viral Immunity
Also see Stress, Autoimmune Disorders, Infection (Bacterial), Infection (Viral)

The immune system is actually comprised of various byproducts created by the proper function of various bodily systems and organs. Unlike the body's nervous system and cardiovascular system, the proper functioning of our immune system hinges on optimal functioning of our physical, emotional and mental processes.

Optimal immune system health is critical and essential for effectively fighting invaders that cause disease, debilities and death. Strong immunity battles cancer, fungi, bacteria, parasites, viruses and toxins that otherwise would weaken the body.

With optimal immunity, the whole body and organ systems work en tandem to protect themselves, necessary and committed allies for the person's entire life.

A tremendous interconnection of the body's various chemical processes defend against disease and sickness. This way a strong immune system serves as the foundation of good health. Things can and do go wrong when, as the age-old saying proclaims, "a house divided against itself will not stand.

Although all this might sound complicated, it's actually easy for average people to clearly understand upon learning about the basic components of healthful immunity.

Weak Immunity Symptoms

Experienced doctors immediately recognize potential immune system impairments upon observing continual allergies, frequent colds or flu, constant or persistent inflammation, slow healing, recurring infections, or chronic diarrhea. Viral infections HIV, HPV, EBV, HSV I and II, and HHV-6 all weaken immune function.

Immune System Enemies

For the most part, people with damaged immunities usually neglect their own health, or they're overexposed to harmful toxins. Severe or catastrophic immune system damage can occur when the body strives to battle a massive invasion of antigens that are extremely difficult to fight. Brief, intermittent, consistent or prolonged exposure to toxins exacerbates a weakened immune system or triggers the problem. Adverse behaviors such as drugs or excessive alcohol or caffeine serve as additional stumbling blocks, blocking the pathway to what otherwise might be optimal health. Negative lifestyle habits, an inadequate diet or failing to take adequate supplements also can weaken or obliterate immunity. Chemotherapy (full dose) and radiation therapy always weaken immune function.

Immune System Boosters

The best, most effective strategy to re-fortify or boost immunity involves a whole-body approach that stimulates the thymus and addresses toxins—all while improving hormonal and chemical imbalances. The best basic strategy involves eating well, mainly whole foods, antioxidant crops and meals that avoid sugar, alcohol and caffeine. Many volumes of highly detailed books could be written on this vital topic. Yet the essence can be easily summarized by understanding that:

Lifestyle: Improve or bolster your sense of well being by getting plenty of love, laughter and sleep.

Balance: Reduce stress, lower caffeine and take DHEA supplements to optimally balance the functioning of thyroid-adrenal activity and hormones.

Avoid: Stop smoking and limit drinking.

Cooking: Refrain from overcooking natural foods, because overheating destroys vital enzymes and microorganisms including "good bacteria" that help the digestive tract.

Natural: Boost and fortify the production of white blood cells that fight invaders by taking maitake mushroom extract. This forms beta-glucans, stimulating the growth of white blood cells due to a sugar-protein complex, thereby fighting cancer and enhancing immunity. The specific white blood cells include "B" cells, "T" cells and "natural killer cells.

Supplements: These should include Vitamin C, and herbs like mistletoe extract, olive leaf extract, goldenseal, Echinacea, Panax ginseng, colostrum, reishe, noni juice, moringa juice, beta glucan, arabinogalactan, olive leaf extract, and liquid colloidal silver.

Diet: Take green drinks comprised of Spirulina, Chlorella and maca. Eat antioxidant foods including carrots and citrus fruit. Eat foods deemed high in fiber, antioxidants and nutrients. With equal urgency, while avoiding processed foods and artificial ingredients, your meals should be low in sugar, salt, carbohydrates, starch, cholesterol and saturated fats. Also, eat ample amounts of "super foods" packed with optimally balanced ratios of essential nutrients. These include kale, maca, bee pollen and olive leaf extract.

Infection (Bacterial)

Also see Urinary Infections, Infection (Viral)

Standard allopathic medicine is losing its overall battle against bacteria, as natural medicines provide power against such infections in a totally different realm. To understand this, first keep in mind that bacteria are single-cell organisms—the smallest microscopic level where life can occur. Bacteria replicates or "duplicates" one cell at a time, but many cells can grow en mass at a huge rate.

Upon invading the human body, some microorganisms have taught themselves how to fool or deceive common antibiotics used by standard medicines. This condition, in turn, has increased overall danger from bacterial infections because the single-cell organisms are "learning" or "teaching" themselves how to create maximum damage.

In fact, bacteria have the ability to mutate into many forms that are resistant to antibiotics. As a result, people need to do their utmost using natural methods to fortify their own immune systems, sharply increasing the probability that their bodies will successfully battle such invaders.

Disturbingly, bacteria engage in their initial attacks by taking advantage of weakened immune systems. To understand how to decrease this danger, people need to understand that bacteria are not viruses. Bacteria are living organisms. The lowest forms of life are viruses, which enter, damage and change the body's cells, sometimes so radically that they sometimes change the person's DNA, our unique biological signature.

Adding to the complexity, our bodies have many kinds of bacteria, some "good" at assisting our cells and digestion, and some "bad," wreaking havoc on health. The good are called probiotics—the bad are pathogens.

Bacterial Infection Causes

The vast majority of bacterial infections involve weakened immune systems. For this to occur, the person must come into contact with dangerous bacteria. Then, if the individual's immunity is weakened or compromised, the bacteria try to seize an opportunity to create damage. Yet people with strong immune systems can escape danger even when attacked by bacteria that wrecks the health of another person with weak immunity.

Urinary or vaginal bacterial infections hit women prone to the condition, usually due to dieting deficiencies, bathing in bacteria-rich water, soiled clothing, hormonal imbalances or sexual contact that transmits harmful bacteria, viruses, parasites and fungal infections.

The potential for harmful bacteria growth to accelerate within the body increases within the bodies of those who eat too many sugars, or whose bodies are more acidic than alkaline. Nutrient-poor diets, inadequate sleep or stress compound the problem.

Additional Considerations

Only take prescribed pharmaceutical antibacterial medications when absolutely necessary. These products promote systematic yeast overgrowth and digestive issues.

Bacterial Infection Treatments and Prevention

Hand washing and behaviors that advocate "proper hygiene" decrease gastrointestinal infections by 80 percent. Similar behavior decreases by at least 50 percent the probability of contracting both viral and bacterial infections.

Avoid sugar, which attracts bacteria while muting the immune system. The most beneficial antifungal and antibacterial remedies topically applied include extracts like the oils of garlic, silver, tee tree oil and oregano. Take supplements containing devil's claw, oregano oil, Echinacea, Probiotic cultures, garlic oil, Pau d'arco tea, and olive leaf extract.

Colloidal silver often proves extremely powerful at battling horrific or seemingly unbeatable bacterial infections, such as yeast infections caused by Candida and even potentially fatal pneumonia suffered by people with AIDS. Never use colloidal silver for extended periods, and only use the non-chemical type of colloidal silver along with golden-colored silver, purchased from a reputable source

Other natural minerals and herbs provide various benefits and potential issues. Echinacea stresses the immune system so only use intermittently. When taking goldenseal as an antibiotic maintain the schedule provided by a practitioner of natural medicine, regularly until the entire recommended total is gone. People suffering from adrenal exhaustion should avoid large doses of Vitamin C. But those without that condition who experience bacterial infections should take this vital nutrient.

Infection (Viral)

Also see Infection (Bacterial), Colds

Essentially microscopic parasites, viruses live off of other organisms, benefiting from the weaknesses of those victims. People with weak immune systems are more susceptible than individuals with strong immunity. Persons with weakened immunity due to adverse lifestyle habits or from neglecting their health are essentially sending a wide-open invitation to harmful and potentially dangerous viruses.

People lacking viruses are more prone to good health, while people with these invaders suffer a greater probability of poor health.

Virus Definition

Viruses are the lowest forms of living organisms. Technically, viruses reproduce themselves in the cells of living organisms, comprised of molecules or particles—damaging the cell, and thus ultimately the person. Scientists admit they lack a single universal method of completely eradicating viruses, which are difficult to eradicate because they become dormant for months or years, and only resurface when the body's immune system is compromised.

Antiviral Treatments

Make your body an unwelcome place for viruses by taking high doses of digestive enzymes as recommended by a medical professional. This helps clean excess waste from the lower bowel where viruses often multiply. Some viruses essentially "burrow into" the body, essentially becoming dormant (i.e. shingles and hepatitis I and II) until adverse foods and lifestyle habits awaken them from that state. Poor diets, smoking, drugs, alcohol, sleep issues and a negative mindset are among contributing factors.

Keep your immune system strong serves as the best defense

against viruses. People with such characteristics often remain "free" of such invaders. You can take antiviral supplements daily to boost immunity. With equal intensity, everyone should avoid sugar, toxins from food and the environment, additives, excess alcohol, stress and smoking.

For ultimate antiviral protection, take skullcap herbs, Saint John's wort and Echinacea. Get plenty of sunlight and exercise daily. Boost the immune system by regularly eating health-forming, nutrient rich foods and olive leaf extract.

Zinc is a formidable weapon against nasal discharge, coughs and common cold symptoms. Supplements also should contain Citricidal grapefruit seed extract, Vitamin C, lysine and N-acetylcysteine or NAC, and colloidal silver from a reputable source rather than homemade.

Inflammation

Anti-Inflammatories

Also see Joint Pin, Arthritis

Many types of illnesses, lifestyle habits and diseases can generate inflammation—an adverse symptom, sometimes from a potentially fatal condition. The many diseases, illnesses and conditions generating inflammation include multiple sclerosis, Lou Gehrig's disease, arthritis, Alzheimer's, heart or arterial disease and Parkinson's disease.

Inflammation Causes

Most of the time inflammation stems from the autoimmune system accelerating into overdrive, used by the body as a protective mechanism to form heat while also surrounding an injury. White blood cells strive to fight infection after racing to the site, with inflammation possible in any part of the body.

Digestive problems sometimes trigger chronic and dangerous inflammation. The immune system's activity skyrockets into overdrive, generating intestinal inflammation while battling bacteria, viruses and parasites, or responding to allergic reactions.

The most common offenders in generating intestinal inflammation include dairy, sugar, wheat, simple carbohydrates, polyunsaturated oils and trans fatty acids. Pain sometimes erupts throughout the body as inflamed tissue presses on vital organs, nerves, muscles, tendons or bone.

Additional Considerations

Avoid dangerous anti-inflammatory drugs that generate many adverse side affects on the stomach, liver or kidneys, called non-steroidal anti-inflammatory drugs or agents (NSAIDs).

Inflammation Treatments

Prescription drugs sometimes cause inflammation, and avoid sugar and starches that can worsen inflammation. Also, drink lots of water because inflammation worsens in people who are not hydrated.

Within healthy people optimal hormone levels regulate or keep inflammation in check. Omega-3 fatty acids from almonds, walnuts, tuna and wild salmon provide help. People who dislike fish can take fish oil supplements.

Eating unhealthful balances of proteins, carbohydrates and oils can generate a negative body response that creates unhealthy or dangerous inflammation. This can curtail or block the body's essential healing and invader-fighting processes.

For optimal results take large doses of enzymes under the guidance of a health care professional. Comprised of life-sustaining proteins, enzymes accelerate the body's chemical reactions, a process which under healthy conditions can generate essential body functions like reproduction, breathing, digestion, nerve health and growth.

When used correctly, particularly under the guidance of a health care professional, enzymes prescribed in supplement form can boost or fortify various bodily functions. This factor is so powerful that pain and inflammation often subside upon taking enzymes on an empty stomach. To remove waste from the circulatory system, use DHEA or "dihydroepiandrosterone."

Other healthful natural remedies hinge on the fact that the Standard American Diet contains substances that lead to inflammation. Among herbs, supplements, lifestyle changes and foods helpful in preventing or reversing these inflammation problems:

Curcumin: Derived from yellow pigment within the turmeric herb, this lowers inflammation by promoting healthful circulation.

Berries: Many varieties help fight inflammation with polyphenols.

Quercetin: Derived from onions, grapes and garlic, this anti-inflammatory can be taken in supplement form.

Arnica: Applied topically or taken orally, this can heal minor inflammatory wounds.

Vitamins: The natural and essential vitamins A, C, and E protect the body from dangerous free radicals while preventing inflammation and keeping joints healthy by boosting antioxidant levels.

Devil's Claw: Containing the same substance used to make natural aspirin, white willow bark, this should be in anti-inflammatory supplements with turmeric and ginger.

Insomnia

Sleep Disorders

Also see Restless Leg Syndrome

Chronic sleep disorders can cause varying health problems, accelerate aging or even lead to early death. The bodies and minds of most people fail to function at full capacity if they fail to get an average eight hours of restful, undisturbed nightly sleep.

Negative or disturbed sleep habits can worsen the mood,

impair immunity, and disturb muscle tone. Long-term chronic sleep disorders sometimes generate dangerous hormonal imbalances while any effort at scheduled rest goes off kilter.

Insomnia Causes (Biochemical)

Eating too close to bedtime and having an overly acidic body disturbs or prevents healthful sleep patterns. Chronic or periodic hormone imbalances, a failure to exercise, arthritis pains, illicit drugs, prescribed pharmaceuticals, and diseases like chronic fatigue syndrome and fibromyalgia can disturb or prevent sleep.

Insomnia Causes (Neuro-Emotional)

Anxiety, stress, grief, depression, "thinking too much" and other factors caused by emotion also hamper or prevent rest, disrupting essential sleep patterns. Sudden or horrific events that disturb the psyche, commonly called "post traumatic stress disorder" sometimes impairs the mind's ability to rest—sometimes many years after the occurrence.

Insomnia Treatments

Numerous natural, non-drug remedies effectively correct sleep problems. Among them:

Create: Try to develop a dream, rather than mentally focus on a worry or issue.

Napping: At midday, take 15- to 30-minute power naps.

Foods: Avoid chocolates, coffee and soft drinks containing caffeine, and steer clear of the artificial sweetener aspartame that may curtail sleep.

Drink: Enjoy a strong tea or "decoction" containing chamomile, kava kava herb, skullcap, valerian root, and passion flower.

Cleansing: A lengthy cleansing that use herbs recommended by a herbologist or homeopath can battle or kill sleep disturbing parasites. Herbs effective in killing parasite eggs include cloves, wormwood and walnut hulls.

Body Work: A massage, or a deep bodily tissue manipulation from a chiropractor, can reduce or eliminate deep-rooted tension that wreck or prevent sleep.

Mental Health: Relax the body and mind and thereby induce the probability of sleep with natural anti-depressants, particularly kava kava, Saint John's wort, SAMe and 5-HTP

Non-Traditional Medicines: Some health experts believe reflexology, acupuncture or acupressure can help improve or induce sleep by resetting the body's natural internal clock.

Hypnosis: Some practitioners of natural medicine say that self-hypnosis can help relax the body into a state conducive to deep, restful sleep.

J, K & L

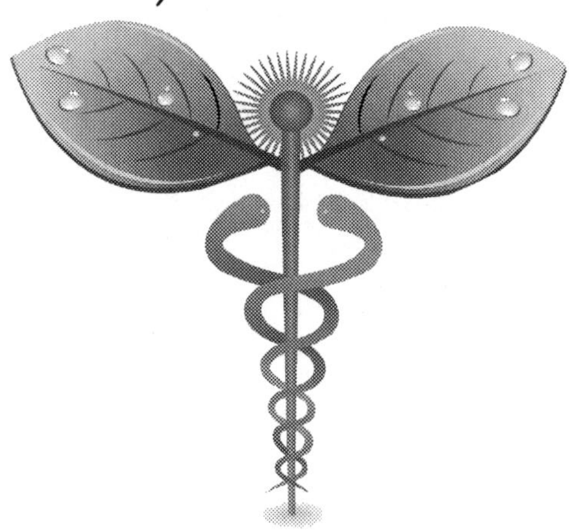

Jet Lag

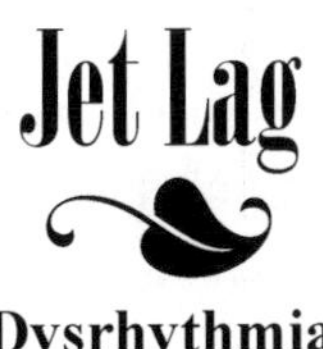

Dysrhythmia

Common "jet lag" symptoms when arriving at a travel destination include everything from an inability to fall asleep to an immediate desire to go straight to bed for rest. Some jet lag suffers feel moody, overly and continually tired, or ill.

Occasionally suffering from "brain fog," while experiencing jet lag some people become unusually moody or feel disoriented, unable to concentrate. Adding to these woes, some individuals lose their appetite, suffer nausea, have headaches and achy joints often due to dehydration—and also complain of diminished libido and energy levels.

Jet Lag Causes

Amazingly, more than 100 essential body functions can get disrupted when a person changes time zones. A recovery period of nearly one week reportedly is typical for people traveling west across five time zones, while for unknown reasons the situation is even worse among individuals going east. Potential factors often cited range from changes in the cycles of light and dark (circadian rhythm), disrupting the body's natural rhythms that regulate eating and sleeping. Additional factors include excessive drinking, stress and dehydration while traveling.

Jet Lag Treatments

For best results, before bedtime take 1.0 to 3.0 milligrams of melatonin, a natural sleep-regulating substance. Also, to accelerate the body's ability to adapt to a new environment, take ginseng and valerian root.

Before, during and immediately after any stage or leg of travel, drink plenty of water to keep the body adequately hydrated. Pure water is by far the most effective for hydration, while juices and decaffeinated tea also can help. For best results, avoid icing drinks, because doing so pulls blood from your extremities as the body strives to warm the stomach.

Other helpful strategies include: taking a 6C dose of homeopathic Cocculus and ginger within ten minutes of boarding a commercial airliner; continually drink pure water every half hour until urinating during the flight; starting a few days before the scheduled departure, go to bed up to a half hour before your usual time; and avoid alcohol, coffee and carbonated beverages.

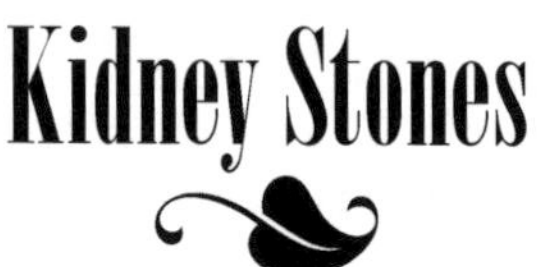

Kidney Stones

Gravel / Renal Calculi

Amazingly, even worse symptoms can occur than the famously horrific and debilitating pain caused by kidney stones. Sometimes as small as a grain of salt or larger, comprised by crystallized minerals, kidney stones can result in fever and blood in the urine and extreme pain while lodged in the ureters. These tubes comprised of smooth muscle fiber propel urine from the kidneys to the urinary bladder. Pain also can be transferred to the lower back, the groin on the same side (ipsilateral).

Kidney Stone Causes

In most cases, kidney stones form when water or other inorganic sources combine with cholesterol-binding inorganic calcium found in dairy products. Tap water high in calcium deposits often impose a major risk. Among other causes are dehydration, gout, excess salt or sugar, purine-rich foods like dried beans and sardines. and drinking too many soft drinks containing phosphoric acid. Never eat excessive amounts of acid-forming proteins. Gout is often a contributing factor among people suffering from that condition or those with a family history of such afflictions. Amazingly, too much consumption of too many specific natural foods or beverages containing oxalic acid can generate kidney stones. These potential offenders include coffee, chocolate, black pepper, wheat bran, spinach, beets, rhubarb, tea and strawberries.

Kidney Stones Treatments

On a steady, regular and consistent basis drink healthful amounts of water good for lessening the severity of kidney stone episodes and preventing such occurrences. Kidney stones sometimes dissolve when interacting with ingested kombucha mushrooms.

Apple cider vinegar can generate amazing results in eliminating kidney stones, and many people proclaim the effectiveness of a weed commonly found in Brazil, puebra pedra, hailed as a fantastic stone breaker. Vitamin C is deemed effective in other regimens, such as a daily 1,500 milligram dose along with 50 milligrams of Vitamin B6.

One of the best remedies often prescribed by homeopaths is comprised of the long silky strings from ripe corn kernels. Called "corn silk," this helps the urinary tract while serving as an excellent diuretic. Corn silk also helps block the kidney stones from irritating or damaging sensitive nephrons within the kidneys. Other helpful remedies include gava root, organic juice and black cherries.

Laryngitis

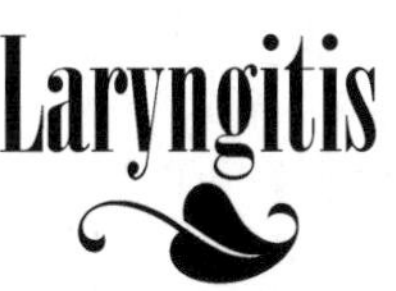

Hoarse Voice

Also see Infection (Viral), Candida, Colds, Infection (Bacterial)

Some people suffering from laryngitis are at least temporary unable to speak, or their voices become gravely, raspy or hoarse.

Laryngitis Causes

A variety of adverse health conditions can cause laryngitis, particularly pneumonia, colds, bronchitis and the flu. Bacterial infections usually serve as an underlying trigger. Allergies, various other illnesses or excessively screaming for extended periods are additional culprits.

Laryngitis Treatment and Prevention

Natural soothing lozenges and throat sprays often provide the best protection and remedy. Either natural or homemade, the most effective ingredients usually include grapefruit seed extract, propolis, Saint John's wort, and liquid Echinacea. Some homeopaths recommend juices comprised of beet, celery, apple, carrot and pineapple.

Liver and Gallbladder Health

Fatty Liver / Gallstones / Liver Cleanse
Also see Obesity, Candida Albicans, Colon and Intestinal Health, Hepatitis

Far too many people abuse their livers, either ignorant of or ignoring the fact it's one of the body's most essential organs. Healthy livers effectively and continuously remove potentially dangerous toxins and other impurities from the body. This process helps the digestive system while providing an optimal process eliminating waste from the person.

Yet severe health issues can erupt when a liver becomes hampered or damaged due to excessive consumption of drugs including alcohol, or if the person regularly eats far too much food—particularly meals loaded with toxins and artificial preservatives.

When the liver becomes unhealthy, harmful wastes build up in the blood and intestines. Similar lifestyles and adverse foods also force the gallbladder to generate potentially painful, dangerous and sometimes life-threatening gallstones. These stones sometimes occur if the liver, the gallbladder or both organs simultaneously become clogged with blockages—sometimes including a backup of bile.

While women are affected most, large numbers of adults experience gallstones, which range from extremely small to golf ball-sized. The problem is so prevalent that gallbladder surgery is among the most common operations performed in the United States.

Symptoms

Some of the most noticeable symptoms include right upper abdominal pain following a fatty meal, dark-colored urine and a yellowing skin called "jaundice." Sufferers of kidney or liver problems sometimes gain weight extremely fast as the body experiences a buildup of fluids that the organs are unable to effectively and efficiently process. Another finding called "fatty liver" occurs when the liver enlarges due to an excessive buildup of ammonia and other toxins. Such chronic liver problems, in turn, can lead to serious diseases including diabetes and abnormal liver enzymes.

Liver Problem Causes

Excessive alcohol prevents the body from effectively removing heavy metals and toxins, and from cleaning the blood. This decrease in liver function can cascade as the organ's health worsens. Poor-quality food, particularly meals loaded with harmful artificial additives and preservatives, destroy or seriously harm the vital functioning of bile production by the gallbladder and the liver. When left unchecked, patient may develop cirrhosis.

Additional Considerations

Available as a dietary supplement and also produced naturally within the body, a synthetic chemical called SAM-e, helps detoxify or clean the liver. Doing this sometimes helps improve the person's mood; toxic-laden livers sometimes lead to depression.

Liver Treatments

Above all, eat generous amounts of antioxidant foods that naturally help the body fight or avoid any buildup of harmful toxins. Besides maximizing efficient cholesterol levels, alfalfa can fortify the liver's bile functions.

To clean the liver and blood, take foods high in alpha-lipoic acid, milk thistle, selenium and certain vegetables—particularly Brussels sprouts, tomatoes, spinach and broccoli.

For pushing toxins from the liver, some homeopaths recommend EDTA. This substance binds to harmful heavy metals, enabling the body to effectively remove those dangerous substances. Used by homeopaths as a chelating agent for more than a half century, EDTA latches on to zirconium, lead, iron, mercury, copper, aluminum, antimony, nickel, manganese, silver, calcium and tin.

You also can benefit from foods containing healthy levels of fatty acids that naturally and effectively push toxins from the liver and the gallbladder. Fish oils work great here, particularly cod liver oil, flaxseed oil, sunflower and safflower oils.

Reduce or eliminate the consumption of liver-damaging foods and substances, such as tobacco smoke, alcohol and drugs including prescription pharmaceuticals and over-the-counter medications—especially acet6ominaphen.

Liver function often improves and the organ becomes detoxified when the person consumes healthy carotenoid crops, particularly peaches, papaya and carrots. Eat healthful quantities of vegetables, fruits and berries having deep colors.

M & N

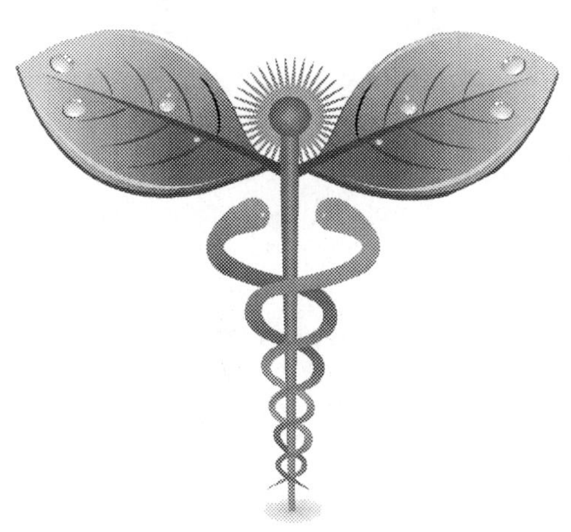

Macular Degeneration

Also see Cataracts, Antioxidants

Particularly among people older than 55, macular degeneration is associated with advanced age. Blindness eventually occurs following a period when the person has an inability to focus vision as the condition slowly destroys the vital central retina within the eye.

Macular degeneration either occurs in "wet" form when scar tissue builds due to an overgrowth of blood vessels beneath the retina, or via "dry" conditions—the most common form—leading to a buildup of debris beneath the retina.

Many suffers of macular degeneration complain of dark spots blocking their field of vision. Objects appear blurred, especially when viewed close up.

Macular Degeneration Causes

Poor nutrition, tobacco and digestive problems are just some of the primary causes. Other triggering factors can include pharmaceutical drugs, excessive exposure to ultraviolet light, environmental toxins, pollution, high blood pressure, digestive problems, and diabetes.

Macular Degeneration Treatments

The good news here is that macular degeneration can be avoided or lessened in severity at least somewhat by taking certain natural measures. Start off by minimizing free radical damage and strengthening cells. A key aspect of this strategy involves avoiding the likely triggers, particularly sugars or foods that convert to sugars, smoking, alcohol, overeating, animal products, unhealthy foods and environmental toxins.

Roll the eyes in simple exercises, varying your focus between near and far. Also, to improve circulation within the eyes, try non-invasive Chelation Therapy.

Benefit from zeaxathin via tangerines, romaine lettuce or corn, or via supplements that also should contain the minerals chromium, selenium and zinc, plus vitamins E and B2, and vitamins A and C with bioflavonoids.

Fruits and vegetables that are orange or yellow generally contain carotenoid antioxidants that help the eyes. Lightly cooked eggs, blueberries and carrots are particularly helpful.

Restore cell strength, as recommended by a homeopath by taking recommended daily doses of the antioxidant astaxanthin.

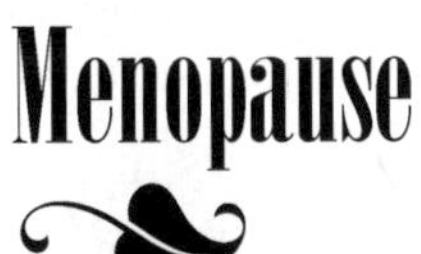

Menopause

Change of Life / Climacteric

Also see Osteoporosis, Hormone Imbalance

Women experience menopause as they age past their natural "menstrual years," when menstruation stops and their bodies naturally and gradually ceases production of the female sex hormone estrogen. This transition often called menopausal signaling, the "change of life" causes problems in many women—but less in societies where females generally lead natural and active lifestyles. So, contrary to a mistaken belief throughout much of society, this transition is not always traumatic on women or on their spouses.

Increasingly erratic, light or short menstrual periods sometimes signal approaching menopause. Amid menopause, a woman's hormones alternatively stop and re-start until stabilization occurs in the individual's natural production of such substances. However, until that natural and predictable leveling-off in hormones occurs, some women experience physical and emotional highs and crashes.

Thus, as their danger of osteoporosis or bone-thinning occurs, some menopausal women become more susceptible to fractures. Adding to their woes are hot flashes, decreased sex drive, water retention and vaginal dryness are common. Some of the worst symptoms can include the urgent need to urinate, increases in yeast infection, depression, poor concentration, palpitations and weight gain.

Even worse, menopausal women can suffer endometrial or breast cancer. Common additional or potential problems include memory loss, muscle pain, itching, insomnia, wrinkled skin and breasts that atrophy.

Additional Considerations

Menopause usually starts between 48 to 52 years of age. It is considered premature if the onset starts before age 40—an extremely rare instance that occurs in about 1 percent of women. Premature menopause can be generated by diabetes, thyroid disease, radiation or chemotherapy, and autoimmune disorders.

Menopause Treatments

Several natural foods, particularly papaya and soy can help address everything from hot flashes and night sweats to helping to bind estrogen receptors. Soy also addresses several menopause symptoms, helping to strengthen bones or to prevent cancers of the uterus, ovaries or breast.

Phytochemicals called "phytoestrogens" from soy, soy products and papaya function almost as if a "surrogate hormone," by binding the estrogen receptors. Some recent research indicates the apparent harmfulness of soy. Yet some practitioners of natural medicines insist that soy only leads to health issues when concentrated or eaten in excessive amounts—and actually may be therapeutic.

Also, pregnenalone also is deemed effective thanks to its ability to transform good cholesterol into the steroid hormones testosterone, progesterone, estrogen and DHEA.

Estrogen replacement therapy was once a widespread treatment, but many researchers now believe such remedies are dangerous if used alone with synthetic hormones. Many doctors once had the mistaken belief that menopause commences when a woman's estrogen levels become depleted. Actually, even after menstruation ends, estrogen production continues intermittently throughout menopause from the adrenal gland sources. In this setting, rose hips and black cohosh along with bioidentical hormonal replacement therapy can be helpful.

Attempts at estrogen replacement therapy fail primarily because such deficiency never completely occurs. In fact, amid menopause many women have excessive estrogen in comparison to progesterone levels.

Mindful of the importance of estrogen replacement therapy, menopausal women have numerous other potentially effective natural treatments that include: Vitamin D3, for minimizing symptoms and preventing osteoporosis; organic calcium to build bones, rather than inorganic calcium derived from bones; and using progestins at the onset of hot flashes to minimize the impact of such episodes.

Menstrual Cramps

Dysmenorrhea

Also see PMS, Muscle Cramps

A surprising one out of every 10 women in the United States suffer from severe menstrual cramps so painful that they're unable to engage in normal activities. Less severe menstrual cramps hit up to four out of 10 women. So, up to one half of all women of menstrual age suffer from cramps, either severe or moderate.

Menstrual Cramp Causes

Progesterone levels drop in all women, forcing the production of hormone-like prostaglandins fatty acids generated by the endometrium. The blood vessels and muscles of the uterus are affected by these prostaglandins. This results in a buildup of metabolic waste products within the muscles, which receive less oxygen. The condition leads to a buildup within the uterine muscles of lactic acid and carbon dioxide, both metabolic waste products. This condition causes the contracting uterine muscles to suffer from increased discomfort and pain. Endometriosis needs to be ruled out in severe cases.

All along, at least half of all women never suffer this way thanks to an ideal balancing of their nutrition. Along with inadequate exercise, frequent contributors include diuretics, coffee, alcohol, cola, chocolate and chocolate amid a low-mineral diet.

Menstrual Cramps Treatments

Among the many effective treatments, strategies and supplements:

Pain control: Use pads instead of tampons, avoid sugar, take a hot bath filled with Epsom salts, drink a cup of chamomile tea every 15 minutes and when trying to relax place a hot water bottle on your lower abdomen.

Vegan: Menstrual cramps may disappear among many women who avoid all types of meat and dairy products.

Natural: Pulsatilla helps balance hormones, thus alleviating or minimizing menstrual cramp pain. Get additional help from 400 IU daily of Vitamin E, and 500 mg of magnesium three times daily.

Gluten: Women sensitive to gluten should avoid all foods containing this substance, which worsens their menstrual cramps. These include oat, wheat, spelt and similar crops or foods made from them.

Night sweats: Use the black cohosh herb and soy products.

Bowel movements: Prevent or address premenstrual constipation by drinking water with laxative herbs (See the Laxatives section.)

Balance: Keep an ideal hormonal balance by using stress-reduction strategies, taking adequate levels of magnesium and calcium, and avoiding high-fat foods.

Teas: Cleanse menstrual blood while boosting healthy menstruation with cotton leaf extract or tea. Important: Only take this for menstruation; for centuries women in South America have used cotton leaf products as "a natural abortive."

Birth Control: Women who use IUDs, or intra uterine devices, should consider avoiding such methods which sometimes worsen cramping.

Tonic: The Asian herb Dong Quai addresses numerous female health issues, loaded with powerful anti-clotting agents and anti-spasmodic qualities—plus vitamins A, E and B12.

Mitral Valve Prolapse

Floppy Valve Syndrome / MVP

Also see heart disease

Mother nature has provided healthy people with heart valves called "mitral valves" that prevent blood from pumping back into the left ventricle. But an estimated one out of 10 people have poorly formed valves that fail to properly close. Most people suffering this type of mitral valve problem have slender bodies. Most cases are diagnosed in women aged 14-30. Thankfully, most people with mitral valve prolapse or MVP function fine with generally normal heart functioning. Yet some of these individuals suffer heart murmurs, rhythmic abnormalities, swollen legs, and fibrillation—conditions that can lead to congestive heart failure and even death. Some patients require surgery, while others are told by physicians "there is nothing that can be done."

MVP Causes

Rheumatic heart disease that can result from severe strep throat, connective tissue issues and collagen problems have been listed as major causes. Some health care professionals believe many instances are inherited, because MVP sometimes occurs in families. Yet nutritional problems or deficiencies are listed by many doctors as the primary cause.

MVP Treatments

First, avoid caffeine which can lead to arrhythmia problems among people with MVP. Secondly, an estimated 62 to 85 percent of people with MVP suffer from magnesium deficiency, according to some studies. Other research indicates that 50 percent to 75 percent of MVP sufferers have Co-Q10 deficiencies. So, take daily doses of magnesium and Co-Q10, preferably under the guidance of a licensed health care professional.

Mononucleosis

Glandular Fever / Kissing Disease / Mono

Also see Infection (Viral), Chronic Fatigue Syndrome

An estimated 19 out of 20 people contract mononucleosis by age 30, commonly called the "kissing disease." Some symptoms pass as a mild malaise, while others suffer a temporarily overwhelming weakness. While in their 30s and beyond, most people never realize they've had mono, perhaps because symptoms generally mimic those of relatively common ailments. The most common symptoms are swollen glands, headaches, fatigue, weakness and sore throats. Some patients develop enlarged livers and spleens.

Most cases occur during adolescence, the age when many individuals begin dating—thus generating this ailment's nickname "the kissing disease."

Some people contract mono without symptoms in early childhood. While "symptomatic" or experiencing symptoms, many people experience symptoms for about two weeks.

Mononucleosis Causes

Usually transmitted via people as they're "asymptomatic"

or not experiencing symptoms, mono is sometimes caused by cytomegalovirus or CMV, or Epstein-Barr virus or (EBV). Although sometimes transmitted via shared needles, utensils or drinking glasses, it's usually transmitted via sneezes, coughs, blood transfusions or saliva.

Scientists estimated that 85 percent of mono stems from Epstein-Barr virus, which attacks the body's natural B cells vital to the immune system. A herpes virus, CMV is listed as the cause of the remaining 15 percent of mono cases.

Mononucleosis Treatments

Perhaps the most important thing to remember is to always take antibiotics while suffering strep throat. Many patients benefit from enzymes, high doses of Vitamin C, a reputable brand of colloidal silver, several days of rest, and pure water, preferably carbon-activated. Failure to take a penicillin derivative may result in rheumatoid fever or kidney disease if a strep throat complicates mono.

Just as important, as your mother may have warned you, "know who you are kissing"—and thus avoid such contact with anyone suffering from a cold or the flu.

Viruses sometimes vary in severity. Patients can suffer the worst symptoms if they get the disease from a person experiencing symptoms, and in some cases even from a "transmitter" who has already suffered symptoms.

The severe and highly bothersome condition of "chronic fatigue syndrome" or HHV-6 sometimes hits people who have been continually exposed to mono—sometimes leading to enlarged livers or spleens. Thus, people with mono should take naps when feeling sleepy to avoid developing chronic fatigue syndrome.

Optimal nutrition helps block or fight mono, particularly nutrient-rich foods like kale, spinach, maca, Chlorella and Spirulina.

Mood Disorders

Also see Energy Enhancement, Anxiety, Depression

Perhaps more than ever many people throughout American society suffer from mood disorders in a vast array of specific conditions. The general categories of these mental issues include anxiety-panic disorder, clinical depression, adjustment disorder and bipolar disorder. As an overall group, these problems are so pervasive that an impressive estimated 44 million Americans suffer from at least some form of mental illness—nearly one out of every six people.

Sadly, many standard-medicine physicians and psychiatrists unnecessarily prescribe extremely dangerous pharmaceuticals to many people suffering from mental illness. Because the vast majority of these drugs are unnatural, some of the worst symptoms generated by antidepressant drugs range from uncontrollable body and facial tics, dystonia, seizures, dizziness, nausea, anxiety, and sexual dysfunction. Thus, rather than helping people, many antidepressants worsen the patients' overall quality of life.

Mood Disorder Causes

While the potential or probable causes are far too numerous and varied to list here in full, many doctors practicing mainstream medicine allied to Big Drug Companies or Big Pharma in the Western world mistakenly blame mental illness on chemical imbalances.

By recklessly prescribing dangerous drugs willy-nilly for almost any mental health issue, for the most part such doctors are striving to use dangerous pharmaceuticals to mask symptoms of mental illness—rather than addressing the underlying problems.

Other physicians strive to address what they consider the underlying causes, neuro-emotional or psychological issues. To say that one method universally works better than the other would be irresponsible. Patients have reported good results from both strategies.

Mood Disorder Treatments

Overall for optimal results homeopaths, standard allopathic physicians and psychiatrists should use both strategies—except preferably without using harmful, expensive and potentially addictive drugs produced by Big Pharma. Instead, doctors should strive to use natural herbal remedies that include:

Exercise and diet: Regularly exercise in moderation, while eating a balanced healthful diet. Generated within the brain, exercise naturally and internally produces the feel-good chemicals or hormones—particularly endorphins and serotonin. These can generate a fantastic natural high without the dangerous side effects of drugs.

French strategy: A study in France indicated that people suffering mental issues following stressful events experienced significant relief after taking an herbal blend of guarana, hawthorn, black horehound, kola nut, passionflower and valerian.

Saint John's wort: Particularly when combined with the natural herb valerian, this is often extremely helpful in addressing moderate anxiety or depression. At least one study indicates that this natural combination is just as effective with fewer side effects than expensive pharmaceuticals such as Prozac.

Mucus

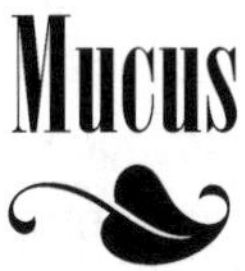

Congestion / Phlegm / Runny Nose
See also Infection (Viral), Colds, Allergies

As a protective measure, the human body generates mucus or the infamous "snotty nose" as a natural, biological effort to remove or fight dangerous bacteria or toxins.

Almost like guards and a moat that protect a castle, mucus strives to prevent such invaders moving further into the upper respiratory tract by protecting membranes close to the body's openings, such as the nose and throat.

When produced on a regular and healthful level while the body is not being attacked and even during such invasions, mucus also serves a variety of essential functions. When moving down the esophagus, food gets lubricated by mucus and saliva as part of an initial phase in the overall digestive process. Within the cervix, mucus helps move spermatozoa toward the uterus while preventing infection.

Yet the body sometimes generates too much mucus when exposed to elevated levels of bacteria or allergens, or when malfunctions occur in the body's natural cleaning mechanisms.

Excess Mucus Causes

Allergic reactions are the most common cause. Milk, chocolate, bananas and apple juice often promotes the formation of mucus even among people without allergies. Additionally, people allergic to these foods often suffer from excessive mucus. Additional common causes include hormones, environmental toxins like pesticides, insecticides, parasites, yeast and bacteria.

Excessive Mucus Treatments and Prevention

Eat organically grown crops and meats. Wash your body and hands regularly to avoid bacterial infections, and refrain from overcooking meats. If necessary, rotate foods to identify allergenic crops or foods. On an empty stomach, take enzymes to digest excessive mucus. Specific natural antibacterial herbs help stop or minimize mucus caused by bacteria and viruses. The best remedy compounds or supplements here contain liquid Echinacea, Saint John's wort, liquid silver, olive leaf extract, and colostrums.

Remove mucus with chickweed, and colon cleanse treatments sometimes effectively address chronic mucus. Gargle at least once daily with one cup of water containing red sage extract. Body-warming herbs like turmeric, cinnamon and cayenne can help.

Muscle Aches and Cramps

Also see Menstrual Cramps / Myalgias

The vast majority of people suffer from extremely painful cramps at least sometime during their lives. The extreme discomfort usually hits the legs and feet, but can occur almost anywhere in the body. Some athletes are among those who suffer this ailment.

Muscle Cramp Causes

Nutritional deficiencies and particularly dehydration are often major contributing factors. Insufficient levels of magnesium and potassium often trigger muscle cramps. Slight calcium deficiencies generate cramps, usually in the legs. The many other potential or probably causes are poor physical conditioning, overextending muscles, extreme cold, low sodium, and overexerting muscles. "Statin" drugs and Erectile Dysfunction drugs (Cialis®) may cause severe myalgias.

Muscle Cramp Treatments

Amid a muscle cramp, relieve the condition while breathing slowly, and by gently and gradually stretching and extending the affected muscle. Regularly using yoga-style stretching techniques are a good prevention method. Relieve spasms and relax the muscle by massaging with natural and healthful oils like chamomile and lavender. Muscle flexibility and superficial blood circulation improve when applying heat. Prevent future cramping by drinking lots of water, stretching regularly, exercising vigorously and doing Pilates, and enjoying plenty of green tea. Stop muscle cramps fast with generous doses of skullcap herb and magnesium citrate with food. Electric vibrators are often helpful.

Nail Fungus

Most nail fungus emerges fast. Yet many instances of this disturbing and sometimes painful condition take many weeks or months of steady, methodical remedies to eradicate. A common easily visible symptom usually includes darkening and thickening of their toenails. For most people the dark spots seem permanent because the people lack details on how to destroy the hard-to-kill fungus which prefers living in dark, damp environments.

Nail Fungus Causes

Fungus usually lives all around us or at the very least throughout most earthly conditions an environment exists for fungi to grow and thrive. Toenails become discolored and brittle when attacked by various fungi such as Trichophyton, which generates nail fungus. Moist or wet socks sometimes serve as contributing factors.

Nail Fungus Treatments

Always wear clean, dry, preferably socks because fungus thrives in moist environments. Wear well-ventilated or open-style shoes, never tight. At both the end and top, file down any nail that hosts fungus. Until the dark spots disappear, rub or apply vinegar or antifungal oil such as tea tree oil, pure pine oil, oregano oil daily or 10-percent solution of Chlorox.

O & P

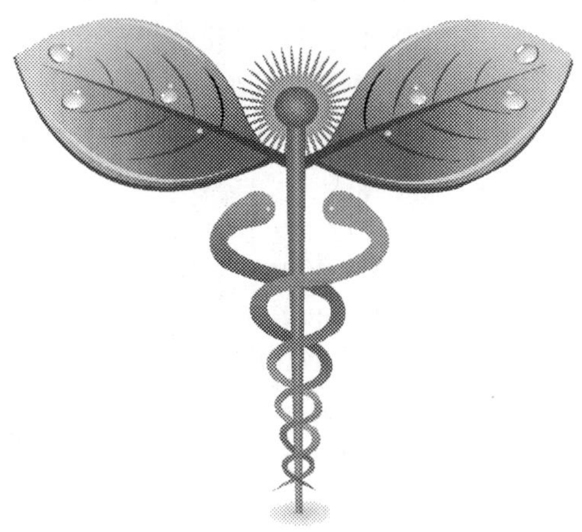

Oral Ulcers

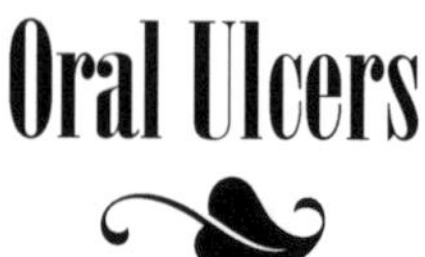

CDanker Sore / Aphthous Stomatitis / Aphthous Ulcer
Also see Cold Sore

When mucus membranes break out in the mouth or lips extremely painful oral ulcers can erupt, but may be misdiagnosed as herpes. The red lesion called a "canker sore" appears after initial burning or tingling. Usually encircled by a white or red border, the sores cause painful jaw swelling.

Even without treatment, the body's natural defenses usually eliminate individual or groups of small oral ulcers within two weeks without negative impact. Even with treatments, however, larger, more painful ulcers can leave scars while taking more than 30 days to heal.

Oral Ulcer Causes

The most common causes include Candida infection (thrush), Vitamin C products including citric acid and ascorbic acid, illness, deficiencies in iron and B vitamins, especially B12, hormone imbalances, gluten intolerance and side effects from chemotherapy.

Oral Ulcer Treatments

Accelerate healing by applying Vitamin E directly to the sore. Attack sores by holding a warm concentrated solution of saltwater inside your mouth, as warm as you can tolerate and for as long as possible. This will cause a sting. Yet that reaction is a positive sign that the solution is cleaning or attacking the infection, while aiding the ability of tissues to clot and contract. Swish the solution near the sore, holding the liquid inside your mouth until it cools. Natural healing will enable the sore to shrink naturally, after a brief expansion period. L-lysine speeds healing along with zinc.

Also take deglycyrrhizinated licorice or DGL in a chewable

tablet form also containing aloe vera gel. Delicate mucus membranes within the mouth should heal thanks to the gel. This chewable can generate healing within three days in three out of every four patients, according to researchers.

Osteoporosis

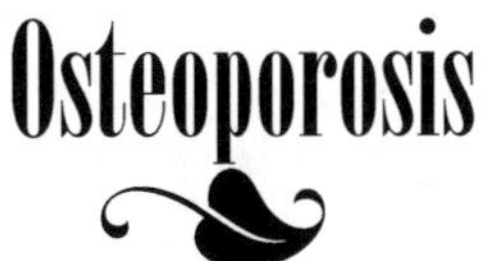

Also see Thyroid Imbalance, Adrenal Imbalance, Hormone Imbalance, Menopause, Osteopenia

Osteoporosis sharply increases the probability of broken bones, particularly among seniors. Bones become fragile, brittle and less dense when osteoporosis strikes, particularly among women who during or after hormonal changes from estrogen loss in menopause hinder their bodies ability to absorb calcium. The problem intensifies as muscles shrink during a person's mature years, making the skeletal structure more susceptible to damage. This condition is preceded by osteopenia or thinning of bones—a precursor to osteoporosis.

Osteoporosis Causes

A leading cause is hormone imbalance caused by menopause, the aging process or from the effects of medical treatments or surgeries. Diabetes, adrenal imbalances, chemotherapy and thyroid problems are other offenders. Drinking sodas containing phosphoric acid or consuming dairy products can cause or worsen osteoporosis.

Osteoporosis Treatments

The best treatment for preventing or addressing osteoporosis is a combination of Vitamin D3, magnesium and calcium.
The good health of much of your body depends on calcium, particularly the bones, muscles, ligaments and cartilage. Yet many

people apparently are unaware that the body fails to assimilate calcium unless magnesium—which enables calcium to enter the bones as nature intends. In fact, without magnesium calcium builds to unhealthful levels within soft tissue and joints.

Homeopaths recommend boron to increase the amounts of magnesium and calcium retained by the body, which otherwise might excrete too much of these essential minerals. Studies indicate bone loss decreases among people taking boron.

Drink ample amounts of water, and benefit from specific herbs via tea or capsules. The best natural herbs for treating and preventing osteoporosis include dandelion root, wild yam, sage, nettle, horsetail, sarsaparilla, alfalfa, chastetree, and black cohosh.

Many people mistakenly believe that cow's milk builds bones, when in fact the opposite is true. Although produced naturally, such liquid actually can threaten health when mixed with cholesterol among mature people. This condition leaches organic calcium from bones while generating kidney stones or gallstones. Among other considerations:

Exercise: Move your body and lift heavy objects within reason, particularly under the guidance of a workout professional. Building strength fortifies bones, as exercise pulls calcium into the skeletal structure.

Fatty acids: Maintain and balance bone calcium via essential Omega-3 fatty acids derived from fish oil, and from essential fatty acids or EFAs prevalent in borage and evening primrose.

Avoid hysterectomy: Never allow physicians to remove the uterus and ovaries unless absolutely necessary. Even among mature women a lack of these organs can lead hormonal changes that generate osteoporosis. Certain drugs and thyroid disorders can lead to this adverse condition.

Progesterone: Unlike synthetic hormones that can generate negative side effects, natural progesterone cream for women increases bone density while also addressing various menopausal and PMS symptoms. The cream works when used daily for at least one month by post-menopausal women, and two weeks monthly for pre-menopausal females in the last two weeks of the menstrual cycle.

Clean water: Drink only clean or filtered water, from which excessive levels of fluoride have been removed. This substance depletes bone strength. Fluoride is found in everything from mouthwashes, toothpaste and chewing tobacco to teas, some wines, snuff, pesticides, topical dental gels, and pots or pans coated with Teflon.

Acidic: Avoid foods likely to make the body more acidic, particularly caffeine, alcohol, protein, sugar, dairy products, fried foods, pasteurized milk, soft drinks, and commercially processed foods. Meantime, eat foods likely to increase the body's alkalinity, particularly wild fish, beans, seeds, nuts and organic, raw leafy green vegetables, and green drinks containing wheat, rye and barley grasses.

Poison Oak/Ivy

Poison ivy and poison oak each generate an irritating sting on the bodily area that comes into contact with these substances. Many people fail to realize that an entire family can suffer these symptoms when pets, children or older family members inadvertently bring or "carry" these poisons into a home environment.

Although generating extreme discomfort or irritation the poison is not life-threatening. The condition should be treated, partly because poison can spread to other areas of the body unless dressed and cleaned.

Poison Oak/Ivy Rash Causes

Embossed in fixed oils the poison takes extensive time to evaporate if at all, while also extremely difficult to wash away. So, immediately and thoroughly wash the person's skin or the pet's fur that has been exposed. Clean the person's clothes as soon as possible.

Poison Oak/Ivy Treatments

Take positive measures to minimize the impacts of rashes, because after that symptom erupts little can be done to stop the poison's impact. Some homeopaths recommend treatments with Jewel Weed, a plant that often naturally grows near stinging nettles, poison ivy and poison oak. Daily until the rash disappears, directly onto the affected area squeeze juice from Jewel Weed leaves.

Among the primary treatments you should perform:

White flower oil: Often used by practitioners of Chinese Medicine, this remedy sometimes stops rashes thanks to the restorative qualities of certain essential oils.

Clorox: Apply the half-strength variety of this bleach to the rash, causing a minor sting that subsides within one minute. However, use extreme care because Clorox sometimes generates disorientation or dizziness. Apply and wash with water and naphtha soap after the Clorox dries.

Natural balms: To relieve itchiness and other symptoms, apply specific natural balms after washing the fur or skin. Acting as an anti-inflammatory, lavender oil helps dry the skin. A soothing mix of baking soda and witch hazel as a paste can soothe inflamed skin while also drying blisters.

Vitamin C: Take this essential vitamin orally, and also combine a Vitamin C powder with water before applying to the rash.

Tea: Dip a washcloth into a tea comprised of two tablespoons of dried chamomile, before rubbing the rash with the wet material.

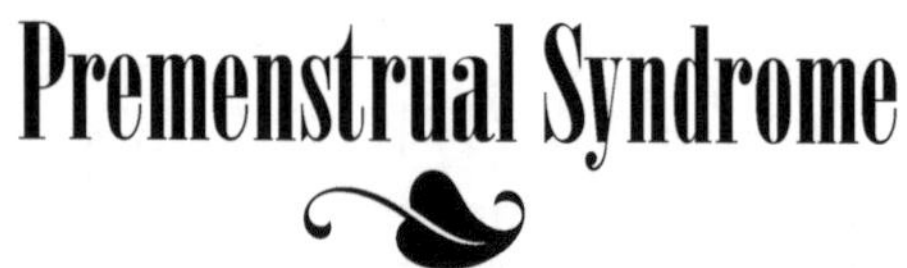

PMS / Periodic Mood Swings / Premenstrual Tension (PMT)

Also see Menstrual Cramps, Cramps, Hormone Imbalance

Sadly and disturbingly, an estimated three out of every four women of reproductive age suffers from at least some degree of PMS. The vast majority of today's doctors and patients strive to address the symptoms of premenstrual syndrome rather than using remedies for the underlying cause. A pattern of various symptoms rather than a disease, PMS generates various adverse conditions that sometimes have a logical connection—but not always.

Common symptoms range from increased fastidiousness, weepiness, dizziness, fatigue and irritability. With similar intensity some women suffer varying degrees of indigestion issues, breast tenderness, backaches, cramping, leg aches, bloating, pimples, nausea, migraine headaches, and skin rashes.

Severe cases sometimes generate suicidal depression. Millions of women start suffering a wide range of mood disorders and physical ailments starting from two to 10 days before menstruation begins. Common life-altering symptoms include depression, bloating, mood disorders, uncontrollable rage, severe pain and insomnia.

PMS Treatments

The best, most effective natural PMS remedies start with effective natural diuretics, especially horsetail herb, strawberries, parsley, watermelon, asparagus and artichokes. While watching sodium intake, and avoiding refined carbohydrates and sugar, the other most effective foods include tomatoes, bananas, potatoes, raw sunflower seeds, peaches, dates and figs. For centuries women suffering PMS in the Andes have used maca root to relieve symptoms..

With similar dedication, PMS sufferers should avoid caffeine, icy or cold foods and drinks, licorice and salt. Among other strategies:

Prevention: Take calcium nightly, when daily meals have included calcium destructors like rhubarb, spinach, chocolate or beet greens.

Magnesium: The vital mineral magnesium often decreases in women shortly before menstruation, so take 500 milligrams of this daily along with 1,000 milligrams of calcium.

Outdoors: Get healthful levels of sunshine, or when such excursions are impossible take 5,000 IUs daily of Vitamin D.

Alcohol: Avoid all types of liquor which can lead to acidic biological environments that damage the liver and deplete magnesium. Avoid caffeine for similar reasons.

Herbs: A wide variety of herbs each relieve specific PMS symptoms. For abdominal cramping, take the Chinese herb xiao yao san and chasteberry. Lessen bodily water retention with Dong Quai. Calm nerves with Saint John's Wort, while 500 milligram daily doses of evening primrose oil serve as a good overall tonic. Take black cohosh herb to counteract, prevent or eliminate night sweats.

Supplements: Some women report that a mix of calcium carbonate and Vitamin B6 helps relieve symptoms. Use niacin to balance B2 and B6.

Prostate Health

Prostate Cancer / Prostate Infection / Prostatitis

Also see Sexual Dysfunction, Anti-Inflammatories, Colon and Intestinal Health

Vital to every man's good health, in direct contact with the bladder and rectal cavity the prostate is the mere size of a walnut when absent of disease. Semen that carries sperm from the testicles is stored within the prostate, which performs the essential task of regulating urine flow. Some scientists believe that every man experiences at least some prostate problems during life, increasing with age after 60.

Disturbingly, an estimated one out of every six men currently or eventually will suffer from prostate cancer, which kills more than 30,000 Americans yearly.

Prostate problems generate a wide range of possible disorders. The common symptoms and warning signs of potentially significant prostate problems include weak ejaculation, a dramatic decrease in ejaculate, and frequent nighttime urination. Some men fail to experience full erections, have difficulty urinating, have decreased libido, and have urine that dribbles despite an urgent sensation.

Prostate Disorder Causes

Infections do not usually generate benign prostate disorders. However, some infections stem from bacteria or viruses contracted via the urethra when sexually transmitted. A prostate that swells due to infection sometimes generates difficulties urinating or painful urination.

Environmental toxins sometimes cause prostate cancer. Some people are surprised when learning that fellatio exposes the prostate to bacteria more than vaginal sex and anal sex. Called "prostatitis," the most common prostate ailment occurs when the organ enlarges, making urination difficult or impossible

The precise cause of all prostate cancers remains unknown. Environmental toxins, inadequate nutrition, genetic factors and hormones are among suspected factors. Researchers believe that men who live sedentary lifestyles, or who eat high levels of sodium nitrate and saturated fat have a higher risk of the disease.

Prostate Health Treatments

Homeopaths have identified numerous remedies in preventing prostate problems, which often are invariably challenging to address in many cases after issues erupt. Such doctors suggest plant-based or "phyto" estrogens.

Saw palmetto can decrease the size of enlarged prostates, aided by a variety of circulation-stimulating and anti-inflammatory supplements, minerals and herbs such as zinc, pumpkin seed extract, curcumin, sage, mistletoe extract, lemongrass, pygeum and sterolins.

Practitioners of natural medicine recommend getting plenty of exercise, engaging in regular sexual activity, refraining from a sedentary lifestyle and taking dietary supplements that contain omega fatty acids, plus vitamins B, C and E.

Colon cleansing can be a good preventative measure, and homeopaths also suggest drinking diet green tea daily while avoiding caffeine, starches, excess alcohol, cigarette smoke, coagulated dairy products, excess sugar and saturated fat. Men also should increase their consumption of nuts, soy, fruit and lightly cooked or raw vegetables. Pomagranate and mixed berries as juices are particularly healthy.

R&S

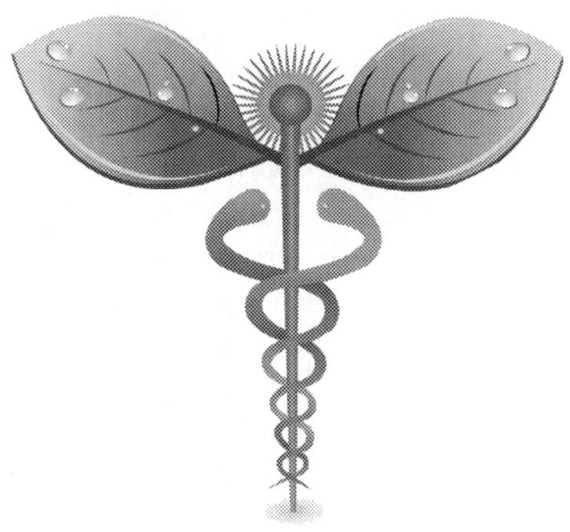

Receding Gums

Imagine putting a taser gun often used for self defense near your mouth and accidentally pulling the trigger. Well, some people who suffer from receding gums report they feel as if suffering an electric shock when touching nerves exposed by the condition.

Doctors report that gums generally recede in tandem with advancing age, but various natural measures can be taken to eliminate, slow or even reverse the condition. Dental nerves can become exposed when gums recede, making the person highly sensitive to brushing and cold or hot food and beverages.

Receding Gum Causes

People who fail to eat adequate amounts of amino acids, vitamins and calcium often suffer from receding gums, while many individuals who take those elements seem to experience less of this condition. Rather than directly impacting the gums, these substances benefit the teeth which serve as the root or base for the gums.

Exacerbating the problem, receding gums provide a continually destructive environment where food particles and bacteria adversely impact the exposed areas. Gums recede further when bone recedes as well.

Far and away, colas serves as the worst culprit as the same substance used to clean bathroom tile, phosphoric acid, corrodes or decays teeth and gums. Certain drugs can accelerate the deterioration of gums and bone.

Additionally, over time a failure to regularly floss and brush can enable the gums to recede and atrophy. Teeth grinding and tobacco use—particularly chewing—can prolong or accelerate such irritation. In a Catch-22 situation, too much or extreme brushing also can force gums to recede.

Receding Gum Treatments

Besides flossing and brushing regularly, be sure to increase your intake of calcium, supplements, Vitamin C, omega fatty acids and herbs like horsetail. Avoid soda, and regularly use hydrogen peroxide or saltwater as a mouth rinse.

Restless Leg Syndrome

Electric Leg Syndrome / RLS

Especially among today's older people who never suffer from restless leg syndrome or RLS, the symptoms sound like a bad plot from a 1950s B-grade horror film. Yet obviously having legs that seem as if they're mysteriously electrified is no laughing matter to people suffering from this bothersome, life-altering and disturbing condition.

The legs feel as if electric-charged with seemingly uncontrollable energy, particularly while lying down or trying to sleep. This disturbs or destroys the ability to sleep in many patients. In some sufferers the legs continually jerk while trying to go to sleep or even when fully asleep.

Particularly when such people refrain from seeking medical help, their legs continue having uncontrollable and relentlessly disturbing energy.

RLS Causes

The exact cause seems just as mysterious to today's scientists as the symptoms would to doctors during a cheap mid-20th Century movie. Yet some researchers blame apparent iron deficiencies, while buildups of lactic acid might also be a contributing factor. Emotional components might play a role as well.

RLS Treatments

Using expensive, dangerous pharmaceuticals or tranquilizers to sleep adds a risk of worsening this condition plus a host of adverse side effects. Although doctors have failed to cure RLS, homeopaths have devised natural, non-toxic ways to control or manage symptoms.

Start off by striving to reduce stress (see the Stress section), and take iron supplements. For improved results, foods or herbs featuring trace minerals can help, particularly rosemary, cinnamon, Spirulina, spinach, bee pollen, curry and thyme. Among other strategies:

Movement: Walk or run daily, primarily during late afternoons.

Liquid: Keep the body hydrated by drinking at least 10 glasses of pure water daily.

Stretching: Stretch the body and particularly the legs daily before bedtime, using yoga techniques or standard stretching exercise methods like palates.

Supplements: Take magnesium daily, plus herbs that relax the nervous system such as Vitamin E, calcium, potassium, as Saint Johns wort, hops, skullcap, valerian root, spearmint, cayenne and ginseng. Quinine (tonic) water may be helpful.

Sexual Dysfunction

Premature Ejaculation / Frigidity / Lack of Orgasm
Also see Erectile Dysfunction

An adequate and satisfying sexual relationship between consenting adults is vital to good overall physical and mental health. The release of built-up sexual tensions via orgasm essentially cleans out the spirit, soul, mind and body for great possibilities. Needless to say, some people insist they feel like "I'm in heaven" during and immediately after healthy sex.

Yet at some point in their lives lots of us suffer from varying types of sexual dysfunction, anything from an inability to get erections, vaginal dryness, failing to achieve orgasm, frigidity with a lack of libido, or becoming "oversexed" amid conditions like nymphomania. This can be caused by diseases or medical conditions like diabetes, heart disease, strokes, cancer, neurological illness, and even bipolar disorders.

Sexual Dysfunction Causes

The causes fall into two categories. First, psychological, emotional and mental problems generate issues in sexual functioning. Second, biochemical and physical issues including performance anxiety prevent the body from naturally performing or desiring sexual activity.

The many likely causes impacting either or both of these two categories range from difficulties and trauma experienced from previous sex partners, chronic depression, fear of sex, a lack of knowledge about sex, and self-esteem and self-confidence issues.

Researchers also believe that poor diets also contribute to sexual problems, particularly among people who eat too many food additives, sugars and saturated fat.

Sexual Dysfunction Treatments

Right away upon being diagnosed with sexual dysfunction problems, be sure to keep an open mind about the potential positive effects of natural remedies. The vast majority of sexual dysfunction stems from psychological issues, best addressed by mental health experts. Countless drugless therapies can help, everything from energy work to psychotherapy.

When dietary issues are suspected as an underlying cause, see the Immune System and the Erectile Dysfunction sections of this guide.

Some patients benefit from using tantra, an ancient method or strategy for engaging in sexual contact while continually mindful of the "present moment" of the experience. Engaging in tantric philosophy and exercise can address many sexual dysfunction barriers. Bipolar personalities have a propensity for nymphomania.

Snoring

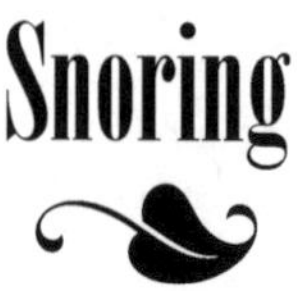

Apnea

Also see Sleep Disorders / Insomnia / Obstructive Sleep Apnea

Snoring impacts an estimated one out of six people, while often disturbing the people they regularly sleep with or attempt to sleep beside. The sound emits from vibrations within areas like the uvula or other fleshy areas within the throat. The specific types of sounds have described as everything from wheezing, rattling and gargling to buzzing or other highly irritating noises.

Snoring Causes

A wide variety of potential causes ranging from mild to life-threatening have been specifically identified. The less serious underlying factors include obesity, loose dentures, nasal polyps, congestion of the nasal or sinus areas, muscle-relaxing drugs including antidepressants that relax the throat and airways, alcohol and eating too close to bedtime.

Advancing age is sometimes a contributing factor as various bodily areas including muscles and skin within the throat become thinner as a person grows older.

Snoring Treatments

Only medical professionals can adequately treat potentially life-threatening snoring, such as sleep apnea which can generate a sudden block of breathing—a condition that can lead to death. Sleep apnea also can lead to a variety of serious long-term ailments ranging from heart disease to lung problems and strokes.

For much less serious instances where snoring imposes a minor inconvenience, homeopaths have developed reliable non-toxic remedies and lifestyle changes. This usually entails losing weight, and avoiding late-night meals. Among other strategies:

Cleanliness: Keep your sleeping environment "dust free," because dust, dander, mold and similar intrusions hamper or block free-flow within the body's airwaves.

Patterns: Go to sleep and awaken at similar times daily. Always sleep on the left side.

Airwaves: Immediately before sleep time, blow your nose to clean air passages.

Position: Sleep on your side instead of the back. Taping a golf ball to your back or arranging pillows in that area prevents sleeping on your back.

Avoid: Minimize or cut down on alcohol, particularly before bedtime. Avoid late-night meals and overeating. Also avoid mucus-producing foods like wheat, dairy products or foods that generate allergic reactions within your body.

Nose: Nasal strips help keep air passages open.

Humidifier: Keep your sleeping environment somewhat humid rather than dry.

Mucus: See the Mucus sections for how to prevent or minimize the body's production or buildup of this substance, which can block air passages.

Sore Throat

Also see Infection (Viral), Colds, Cough, Infection (Bacterial)

Almost everyone suffers a sore throat at sometime in their lives, many of us seemingly on countless occasions.

Immediately upon the first sign of this ailment start taking natural remedies. Early and aggressive treatment can "nip it in the bud," wiping out a sore throat before it grows, worsens or spreads. Particularly when left unchecked, sore throats can worsen to extreme levels, sometimes threatening or seriously impacting bodily areas like the tonsils.

The initial onset of scratchiness or itchiness at the back of the throat usually indicates an invasion by viruses or bacteria. This often worsens when these invaders are fed when we eat sugar or processed food.

Sore Throat Causes

The flu or common colds sometimes introduce sore throats into the body early in their overall processes. Numerous viruses and even germs like streptococcus can generate this symptom. Environmental issues sometimes disturb or inflame mucus membranes in the throat and larynx. These adverse factors include allergies, screaming too loud, acid reflux, vomiting, secondhand smoke, smoking and arid climates.

Sore Throat Treatments

Never be fooled by over-the-counter remedies which merely block symptoms without addressing the underlying problem. While such drugs might relieve itchiness and scratchiness somewhat, they generally fail to attack any bacteria or virus. Conversely, numerous natural remedies often wipe out sore throats. Among the most effective measures to take right away shortly after the moment a new sore throat is felt:

Remedies: Attack the viruses and bacteria with natural non-toxic antiviral and antibacterial remedies, administered via tinctures or herbs. The best choices often are liquid Echinacea with goldenseal, Saint John's wort, propolis tincture, clove leaf, olive leaf colostrum, and colloidal silver.

Vitamin C: At least every 2-3 hours daily for three to five days, take mega-doses of 2 to 3 grams of Vitamin C.

Soothing: For instances where viruses and bacteria are not the cause, ease the discomfort with anti-inflammatory herbs and honey.

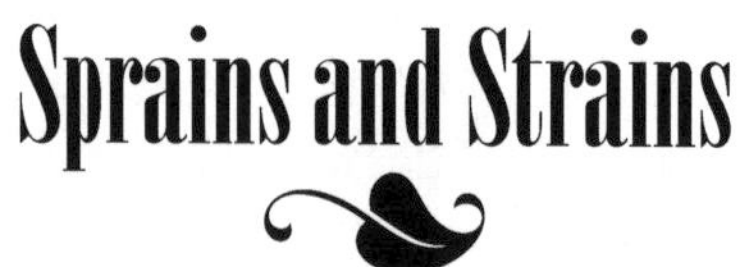

Also see Inflammation

Almost everyone who has lived into adolescence, early

adulthood and into their mature years has suffered from at least some "sprains and strains." Yet many people are unaware that a sprain is different from a strain, perhaps because both conditions generally cause similar symptoms.

Both conditions generate varying degrees of bruising, swelling and pain. Sprains occur due to the stretching or tearing of tendons and ligaments that connect joints to bones. Strains erupt due to the adverse or injurious pulling or twisting of the tendons or muscles that attach muscle to bones.

Sprains and Strains Treatments

Rest the affected limb right away upon feeling a sprain or strain. Avoid putting weight on a leg suffering from such injury. Instead, elevate the affected limb—whether an arm or leg—while applying an ice pack to the joint or muscle. Do this for a minimum 20 minutes. Then use an elastic bandage to immobilize and compress the joint or muscle.

In the process, refrain from cutting off or hinder the blood supply, wrapping the bandage loosely or moderately. Some homeopaths recommend putting steamed anti-inflammatory comfrey leaves on the bandage before wrapping. The leaves accelerate healing while minimizing pain.

To reduce, minimize or prevent swelling that can lead to pain, see the Inflammation section of this guide. Homeopathic arnica is often helpful.

Topically apply homeopathic traumeel for pain. Sit in warm baths filled with Epsom salts amid the healing process. Massages relax and alleviate discomforts in affected areas. Omega-3 fatty acids, bromelain, Vitamin C, and drinks of horsetail tea and comfrey root taken during the healing process can accelerate a return to good health.

Stress

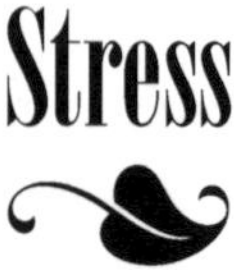

Also see Sleep Disorders, Adrenal Imbalance, Hormone Imbalance

It comes as no surprise to many people that poor health and disease are caused by stress more than any other factor, at least according to many scientists. Stress can potentially influence every aspect of health by causing changes in brain chemistry. Such adverse conditions lead to bothersome, debilitating or life-threatening health conditions that range from cancer, chronic fatigue syndrome and heart disease to backaches, ulcers, insomnia and a wide variety of other ailments. Other potentially dangerous conditions include heart attacks, high blood pressure, cardiovascular problems and stroke.

Usually on a less serious level but extremely bothersome nonetheless, stress also can lead to emotional disorders, sleep issues, fatigue, headaches and various aches and pains. The lengthy list of other ailments or adverse physical conditions that stress can cause include bowel problems, colitis, abdominal cramps, an unusually high number of colds or infections, a weakened immune system, and adverse skin conditions like rashes and itchiness.

Stress Causes

Today's around-the-clock lifestyle coupled with a continual need to survive by performing multiple and seemingly endless tasks can contribute to excessive stress. Adverse effects from illness, poor diets and insufficient sleep also build stress to unhealthful levels. Other contributing factors sometimes include the sudden unexpected death of a loved one, the severe illness of a relative, employment issues, and insufficient income during retirement. Such devastating events catapult stress to extreme levels.

Common everyday tasks also can generate excessive stress. Blood pressure sometimes rises to dangerous levels due to the pressures and impacts that personal responsibilities impose on the body and the mind. These stresses wreak havoc on blood flow to muscles, respiration, metabolism, respiration and heart rates. The body automatically generates these conditions as a response to high-pressure issues.

Most forms of stress result from result from the body's natural biological "fight-or-flight" reactions, which enable mammals including humans to run or fight amid horrific, stressful, or life-threatening situations. Stress becomes a problematic health concern unless such tensions are released. This is a primary reason why exercise, moving the body or engaging in pleasant activities helps people release stress buildup.

Hormones and Stress

Hormones and biological reactions play an integral role in how a person's body reacts to stress. A normally beneficial natural substance called cortisol generally assists the body's functions when released into the bloodstream by stress. Yet the overabundance of cortisol a person experiencing excessive stress can lead to numerous potentially catastrophic or dangerous physical conditions. The worst among these include hyperthyroidism, inefficient immune system, a dangerous belly fat buildup, increased blood pressure and cognitive problems. Excessively high cortisol generated by too much stress adversely effects memory while sometimes leaving the brain open to attacks from toxins. Stress makes people more prone to various diseases including Alzheimer's.

Having fun, exercising, getting regular rest and enjoying sunshine effectively lower cortisol. Yet in a Catch-22 situation, people should refrain from allowing their cortisol levels from getting too low. That condition sometimes generates excess stress, depleting adrenal function. This leads to exhaustion, and may aggravate fibromyalgia or Chronic Fatigue Syndrome.

By having good, clean and healthful fun that leads to laughter and smiles, people can rebalance adrenal function that had been busy making cortisol while producing inadequate DHEA levels. Health care professionals can give tests to determine if specific supplements are needed to change or correct DHEA totals, adjusting those totals in accordance with the various natural cortisol levels. In addition, a health care expert is necessary because DHEA also regulates balances among the body's various adrenal hormones.

Stress Reduction Treatments

Right away stop or minimize any activity likely to catapult stress to unhealthful levels. Seriously consider whether stress-causing activities are worth the effort. Just as important, immediately remove caffeine and other stimulants from your diet. Sugar is another major offender to avoid. Caffeine, stimulants and sugar weaken the adrenal system, creating a biological environment leading to excessive cortisol that puts the body at dangerous stress levels.

Strive to live and work in a quiet, meditative and relaxing environment. Excessive noise and sudden loud sounds shoot the body's stress into dangerous overdrive. Meantime, under the guidance of a health care professional

Eat a healthy diet packed with healthy, nutritious food and herbs like dark colored leafy vegetables, pine bark extract, bee pollen, olive leaf extract.

Therapeutic baths help fill the body with vital life-giving oxygen, relieving stress while enabling the person to better relax and relieve unnecessary tension. Excessive stress shortens the breath, depriving the body of vital oxygen.

Sitting all day without moving the body becomes a recipe for disaster. Exercise or moving the body at the very least can help reverse shortness of breath. Massages and non-traditional medical techniques like acupuncture and acupressure can generate similar benefits. Far-infrared saunas and bio-MATS will help reduce stress.

Stroke

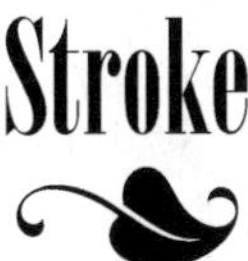

Also see Cardiovascular Health, Heart Disease

Strokes sometimes cause years of catastrophic health problems or even death, but modern medicine has designed ways to effectively prevent and address the condition. The vast majority of strokes decrease brain function by injuring cells within that essential organ.

When a stroke occurs blood flow to the brain usually gets blocked by clotting blood. vessels or causing hemorrhages. Plaque clogged arteries also can lead to the condition, which some people call a "dry stroke" rather than a "wet stroke." Some brain hemorrhages are blamed on substance abuse, high blood pressure and advancing age.

The numerous much-unwanted stroke symptoms include numbness or difficulty of movement on one side of the body, challenges walking or standing, coordination problems, and dysfunction in the speaking voice. Some "stroke victims" experience extreme difficulty swallowing, talking, walking and moving. Lay people call this a "vegetative state."

Initial symptoms immediately following a stroke also can include numbness, loss of hand coordination, cognitive problems, tingling, severe headaches, and even seizures.

Stroke Causes

Doctors list the primary causes as having a type-A personality, stress, high blood pressure with excessive amounts of "bad" cholesterol, and arterial fibrillation with arterial thrombo emboli. Diabetes and both benign and malignant brain tumors may cause strokes.

Stroke Prevention

Scientists say that you can cut your risk of stroke by 50 percent by taking omega-3 fatty acid found in certain fish, particularly salmon, and also found in supplement form. Besides preventing strokes, omega-3 fatty acids as well as decreasing the likelihood of dementia. Taking this essential substance also helps counteract its loss within the body caused by advancing age. Additional benefit comes from the fact that these acids reduce the likelihood of platelets aggregating within the blood; when left unchecked this condition can lead to stroke or heart attack.

Additional prevention strategies involve losing weight if you are obese, getting plenty of exercise and minimizing stress. (See the Stress section of this guide.) Among other primary tips:

Avoid: Eat less or totally cut your intake of sugar, starches, caffeine, harmful drugs, and head trauma.

Red wine: People who drink alcohol should drink small or moderate amounts of red wine, which contains quercetin, and resveratrol that helps reduce stroke risk.

Potassium: Get more of this vital substance from pure cocoa, onions, ginger, bananas, parsley and garlic, which all help reduce blood pressure. Take ginger via extract, teas or food.

More aid: Boost brain circulation with ginkgo biloba, help the heart and arteries with hawthorn berries, and control blood pressure with turmeric.

Stroke Treatments

Get medical attention as fast possible if you know or suspect that you have suffered a stroke. For best short-term results for dry strokes and to minimize damage, some health professionals recommend that you should have the physician give you anticoagulants. Best used within a few hours after the stroke, this helps boost vital and essential oxygen to the brain. Optimal results occur when used shortly after the stroke has temporarily hampered critical blood flow to the brain. Other anti-platelet drugs are now available.

According to researchers, Coumadin is so powerful that it actually helps normalize brain energy metabolites when administered with acetyl-L-carnitine. For the patient's long- and short-term recovery this can make a tremendous difference.

Other potentially effective after-stroke treatments are DMAE, bromelain, Nattokinase®, and Poly-MVA.

Sunburn

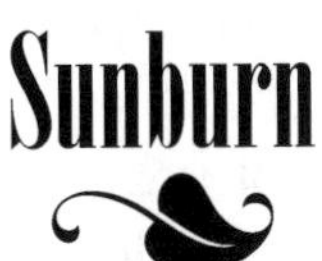

Also see Burns

Often ignored by many people throughout society, scientists often warn that earth's critical ozone layer has gradually and steadily being depleted by carbon-based pollutants. This increases the exposure people have worldwide to extremely harmful ultraviolet rays or UV, which sometimes can lead to cancers many months or years after exposure.

Sunburn Prevention

Minimize excessive sun exposure, wear hats and use creams listed as having high protection against ultra violet rays. Overall, at least some sun exposure is necessary for overall good health, the body uses sunlight to internally generate essential Vitamin D.

Nonetheless, people everywhere need to take precautions from excess sun exposure, particularly if living in a sunny area or vacationing. Contrary to a popular but mistaken belief, dark-skinned people face perhaps just as much danger as people with light skin. Besides UV from the sun, skin damage also can erupt from sun-tanning salons or even high-power lamps for industrial use.

Mother nature usually removes the most painful sunburn symptoms within a few days, while overall recovery for mild to moderate cases can take up to a few weeks.

Sunburn Treatments

Beware of the fact that soaking in water too much can dehydrate the skin, a condition that impedes or slows healing. Use potato pulp or raw plantain to hydrate the skin.

To replenish vital bodily fluids while addressing blisters and swelling, drink lots of water while suffering from sunburn, ideally at least eight 8-ounce glasses daily. Accelerate and promote healing by topically applying Vitamin E cream preceded by aloe vera gel starting after pain subsides. For improved results, fortify the aloe vera gel with lavender oil or calendula. Promptly soothe the heat by generously and frequently spraying carbon-activated water on the affected area. Apple cider vinegar sometimes works if such water is not available.

T&U

Thyroid Imbalance

Goiter / Hyperthyroidism / Hypothyroidism / Iodine Deficiency
Also see Hormone Imbalance, Adrenal Imbalance, Chronic Fatigue, Energy Enhancement

Various critical and life-altering diseases can occur when the thyroid becomes overactive in producing too much hormone, or under-active in generating inadequate levels of those substances. Called "hypothyroidism," the under-active condition is a growing negative health condition that has reached epidemic proportions in the United States. Shockingly, researchers estimate that at least half of all adults suffer at least some degree of under-active thyroid function. The probability of heart problems and increases in cholesterol impose severe dangers. Besides low energy, low ambition, chronic tiredness and obesity, this can result in more colds or flu, reduced sex drive, sluggish digestion weakened immune systems, hair loss, constipation, lowered body temperatures, and menstrual irregularities.

Perhaps just as destructive to overall health, an overactive thyroid—called hyperthyroidism—raises the person's energy as metabolism accelerates. This usually generates adverse excess nervous or "speedy" energy. Weight loss and oversensitivity to heat prove just as disturbing as weakened muscles and sleep disorders. At the mid-central portion of the neck, enlarged thyroid glands sometimes protrude while goiters develop. The many debilitating or bothersome symptoms include shaky hands, protruding eyes, heart palpitation, increased appetite, artrial fibrillation, excessive sweating, heat intolerance, fatigue, and insomnia.

Thyroid Problem Causes

Optimal thyroid health hinges on a delicate balance. Most thyroid problems stem from either too much or too little iodine, which the thyroid needs to produce the important T3 and T4 hormones. The excess or inadequate levels of iodine trigger the thyroid's overactive and under-active conditions.

Adding to the challenges faced by patients and doctors, iodine supplements sometimes become ineffective when the person eats goitrogen foods or salt that blocks this critical substance. Soybeans and peanuts are perhaps the worst offenders here. Foods from the cabbage family also are goitrogens, although you would have to eat massive quantities of that food to be adversely effected.

Additional research puts some of the blame in causing thyroid problems on inadequate water treatment, toothpastes that contain fluoride, selenium deficiencies. Excess caffeine sometimes causes thyroid and adrenal problems. Additionally, imbalances or deficiencies in the adrenal glands and pituitary can adversely impact thyroid function. Thyroid disorders usually fall on the female side of families as a hereditary disorder.

Thyroid Imbalance Treatments

Each person has unique, individualized needs for correcting thyroid imbalances, for which there is no known single universally effective treatment. The best results sometimes occur when properly balancing thyroid function with ideal nutrients, particularly optimal levels of selenium and iodine. All along, patients and physicians should carefully work to modify or adjust such imbalances because accelerating or slowing thyroid activity can mask any underlying issue. Ineffective or inadequate efforts here might address symptoms rather than ideally correcting the underlying cause.

Primarily produced in South America, maca root can help balance thyroid function. Get additional thyroid hormone-balancing benefits from a substance derived from an African plant, the essential oil myrtle. Also, counteract or address the energy problems and adrenal imbalances of hyperthyroidism with ashwagandha, valerian root and motherwort.

Ideal supplements contain rosemary leaf extract, plus vitamins A, D, E, B2 and B3. Ideally, patients should experiment by adjusting wheat germ, brewer's yeast, garlic, walnuts and kelp—all in identifying each individual's ideal balance of estrogen, selenium and iodine. Invariably people with overactive or under-active thyroids should remove high fructose corn syrup and caffeine from their diets, while dramatically cutting back on unsaturated vegetable oils, soybean oils and peanut butter. Replace these foods with cocoanut oil and flaxseed oil rather than saturated fats.

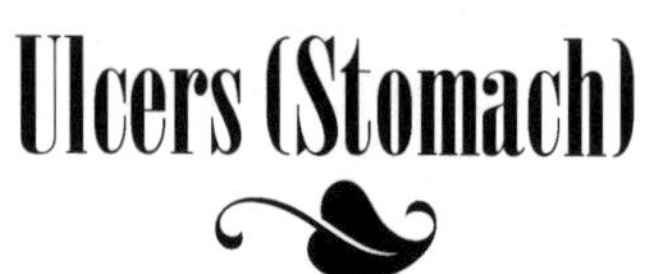

Ulcers (Stomach)

Also see Dehydration, Digestion

Severe cases of stomach ulcers generate vomiting that sometimes contains blood. The less serious but life-altering and bothersome symptoms are weakness, nausea, epigastric pain, bloating and dull stomachaches. This is called "gastritis."

Stomach Ulcer Causes

The vast majority of stomach ulcers, up to 90 percent by some estimates, are caused by eating too much salt, and Helicobacter pylori bacteria. These conditions can lead to gerd and even gastric or esophageal cancers.

Excessive sodium intake sometimes results from eating salt-laden foods like French fries and canned soups. Common early warning signs include dark urine, a darkened complexion, continual thirst, bloodshot eyes and teeth clenching.

The various other likely or potential causes include cigarette smoking, zinc deficiency, excessive secretion of hydrochloric acid sometimes caused by too many NSAIDs like ibuprofen and aspirin. Researchers are still trying to determine why H. pylori bacteria never cause ulcers in some people, while generating the condition in others.

Stomach Ulcer Treatments

Immediately visit or contact your doctor if suffering from

severe symptoms. For both mild, moderate and severe symptoms, start off by getting a thorough medical checkup and a review of your stomach. Eradicating H. pylori bacteria sometimes removes other adverse symptoms, while also enabling ulcers to heal. Other treatment strategies include:

Natural weapon: Taken separately three times daily, benefit from rhubarb root and goldenseal. Allow four to six for beneficial results.

Avoid: Curtail or never use acid-laden chewing gum, which activates digestive juices that worsen ulcers. Some products are okay, however, such as guar gum available in capsule or powder form.

Cranberry juice: Protect and block the stomach wall with this beverage, keeping H. pylori bacteria from that critical area.

Aloe vera juice: When derived from filets, this can heal the stomach's delicate lining. Avoid whole-leaf aloe with contains toxins within the rind.

Garlic: Taken with each meal, this can provide substantial help, particularly when derived from fresh clove.

Slippery elm: This aids digestion while healing ulcers, also addressing Crohn's disease.

Muti-vitamins: Take these daily with zinc that accelerates the healing of ulcers, injury and illness. Chamomile tea also helps.

Get additional benefits from a variety of herbs, particularly turmeric, thyme and cinnamon, plus lemongrass and the essential oils of lemon verbena. If all of the above fails, triple antibiotic therapy becomes necessary for 14 days.

Urinary Infections

Bladder Infection
Also see Candida, Infection (Bacterial), Cystitis, Prostate Health

Hitting far more women than men, urinary tract infections strike an estimated six million Americans yearly. Females are more prone to this condition due to their anatomy, which provide invading infectious organisms less distance to reach the bladder. An urgent or frequent need to urinate, blood in the urine and lower back or flank pain are among the typical initial symptoms. Suffers endure pain while urinating, producing small amounts of urine.

People should seek immediate treatment when first noticing symptoms, which can include pain along the urethra. Early treatment often results in a cure. Patients who ignore early symptoms often eventually suffer fever, fatigue, cloudy urine, serious kidney infections, and possibly sepsis.

Prostate problems can cause urination urge while sleeping, dribbling or straining to urinate. Bacterial infections cause "dysuria," which is among the most common urinary symptoms—meaning painful urination.

Urinary Infection Causes

Different types of physical disorders or health conditions generate separate types of urinary infections between men and women. Particularly when the organ is enlarged, prostate issues are the primary cause of urinary infections among males. Sometimes sexual contact with infected partners generates the condition in men. By contrast, among women the E. coli bacteria generates about 17 out of 20 urinary infection cases. Within female body structures this harmful bacteria can easily move to the urinary opening from the anus—sometimes by wiping themselves following bowel movements from the anal area toward the uretheral region. Also, yeast infections in the vaginal area can lead to urinary infections.

Urinary Infection Treatments

Right when symptoms begin drink a glass of water containing Alka Seltzer, which often within days rids the urinary area of harmful bacteria. Boost these efforts by taking doses from 2 to 3 grams of Vitamin C, taken regularly every 2-3 hours throughout the day.

Eradicate the bacteria with natural herbs, particularly juniper berries, coriander, goldenrod and Echinacea. Natural diuretics can help in tea or capsule form with corn silk, cranberry, uva ursi, horsetail, buchu, nettle, pipsissewa, dandelion, and asparagus.

Safe sex serves as the primary prevention measure, although everyone should remain cognizant of the fact that other potential causes exist. To prevent transferring the bacteria, when engaging in sex, people should refrain from touching the anal area before touching the urinary region.

See the kidney section of this guide on suggestions on how to remedy or prevent the development of kidney stones.

Wash bacteria from the body by drinking lots of clean water daily, helping to prevent bacteria from multiplying as they adhere to urinary tract. Just as important, try to urinate often rather than delaying these bathroom chores. An additional prevention measure involves regularly eating plenty of blueberries while avoiding caffeine

To cure urinary infections, avoid sugar and every day drink at least 64 of water mixed with unsweetened cranberry juice containing natural stevia to enhance flavor.

V & W

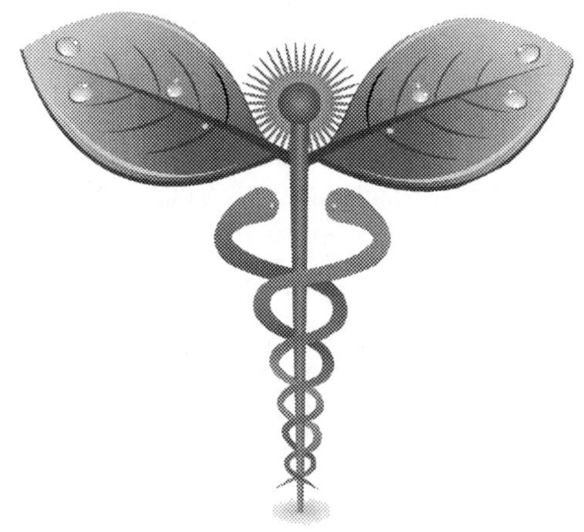

Varicose Veins

Also see Liver and Gallbladder Health

Varicose veins are unsightly, ropey and often painful, primarily striking the legs. Maturing women comprise the vast majority of instances, while men suffer from this ailment less often. Rare extreme cases can lead to severe health issues like deep vein thrombosis, a potentially life-threatening condition. In all cases, enlargement occurs in leg veins due to the failure of leaflet valves which in healthy people prevent the backward flow of blood within those limbs.

Varicose Veins Causes

The extreme difference of occurrences among the genders leads some health care professionals to believe that hormonal issues might be a significant contributing factor. Also, many researchers believe that standing or sitting for extended periods are among primary causes. Blood starts pooling near the feet when standing or sitting for extended periods gradually or quickly forming varicose veins. Pregnancy can aggravate this condition.

Preventing Varicose Veins

Strive to maintain an ideal body weight, in order to avoid becoming morbidly obese. Enzymes like bromelain maintain or energize overall venous health. Keeping active via exercise or moving the body often and regularly can help the body continually maintain healthful blood flow—reducing the potential for the development of varicose veins. Hot, spicy foods that contain garlic, pepper and onions act as a blood thinner. Reduce or stop alcohol consumption, while eating lots of liver-cleansing foods like blackberries, red grapes, cherries, blueberries, cherries, beets, artichokes, milk thistle, gingko, willow bark, and dandelion. Leg massages help overall blood flow.

Varicose Vein Cures

Take plenty bioflavonoid substances with Vitamin C. Many homeopaths recommend horse chestnut herb. Surgical treatment or laser therapy sometimes becomes an option.

Waistline

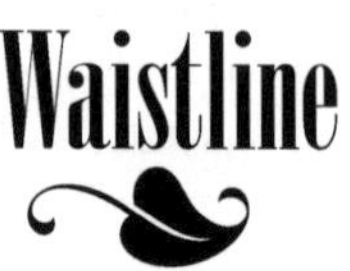

Bloating

Also see Weight (Over), Digestion

Scientists believe that for better overall health people generally should have any accumulated excess weight around the hips and thighs—thus making the overall body appear if pear-shaped. Much less healthful conditions exist and a propensity for more health problems occurs among apple-shaped people. Excessive belly fat leads to a variety of health problems ranging from increases in cancer, cholesterol, heart disease, Type 2 diabetes, along with back pain and strokes. The greater risk here hits men who have far more belly fat than women. All along, women who gain mid-section weight also have a greater probability than medium-size and thin females of developing illnesses like breast, ovary and uterine cancers.

Expanded Waistline Causes

The most famous and likely causes include eating too many calories daily and failing to get adequate exercise while living a sedentary lifestyle.

Lots of people who think of themselves as "fat" actually have a buildup of harmful Candida within their bodies. This condition causes bloating around the face and midsection. Perhaps the most typical symptom indicating excess Candida is a white coating on the tongue. Additional warning signs for Candida include craving sweets, vaginal discharges, fatigue, being mentally confused and swollen eyes.

Huge bellies also might indicate of solid wastes within the colon. Parasites within the colon also cause stomach bulges. Common indicators of parasites include dark circles under the eyes, pale lips, and an itchy "perineum"—the space between the genetalia and the anus.

An over-active thyroid, called "hyperthyroidism" sometimes generates weight loss. In addition, adrenal dysfunction packs on belly fat due to too much cortisol production, before that internal manufacturing slows down too much when the body depletes its energy reserves.

Within Chinese Medicine kidney issues cause a depletion of the body's sexual energy and fear. Kidney problems generate edema where exposure to moisture generates puffiness in the abdomen, around the eyes, and under the skin.

Expanded Waistline Treatments

Some practitioners of Taoist and tantric sex believe that engaging in physical relations while intentionally avoiding orgasm can assist the body in maintaining kidney meridian strength.

Colonics and colon cleanses help remove solid wastes that bloat the abdomen. Numerous natural, non-toxic herbs and certain intestinal flora help minimize Candida. (See the Candida section of this guide.

While eliminating non-nutritious meals, eat more nutrient-dense foods that contain dandelion, Spirulina, Spanish gooseberry, and bee pollen. Keep active enough to sweat at least three times weekly. Use colon- and diet-cleansing strategies to remove parasites from the body. Just as important, avoid mushrooms, vinegar, sweets, bread and pizza, and also fermented foods and alcoholic beverages. Eat fewer meats. Other potentially beneficial strategies include:

Natural Spices: Sprinkle seaweed, particularly focus kelp, and dulse on food to provide the body with enough iodine to help metabolism and thyroid functions. Liberally use tumeric spice.

Natural Cleansing: Flush away fat-generating substances

with raw garlic, cat's claw, and black walnut in extract or capsule form. (See the Constipation section of this guide for more digestive tract cleansing methods and herbs.)

Water: Drinking lots of water daily can help break and flush away excess body fat.

Conjugated linoleic acid: Although rarely known by most people, this amazing substance has shown substantial effects in removing belly fat—particularly among sedentary people.

Diversity: Eat spicy food to invigorate the metabolism, while using chickenweed to remove body fat.

Warts

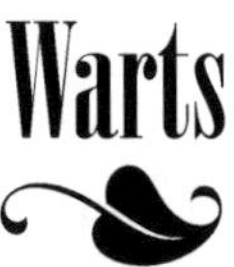

Also see Human Papiloma Virus

Do you remember that age-old wives tale that warns, "If you touch a frog, your hand will soon have a wart?" Well, the good news here is that transfer of warts among different species never occurs. However, there is some essential news about warts, which most typically appear on the hands and feet in cases where humans are involved. Warts are growths, bumps or tumors that usually disappear within a few months. Yet sometimes weeks, months or even years after disappearing warts reappear. Adding to the challenge, warts can travel to different bodily surface areas.

The size and appearance can vary greatly among warts, which emerge alone or in clusters. Clothes and muscle movement sometimes irritate these growths, the severity hinged at least partly on the size and structure of each lesion.

Usually yellow, gray, grayish-black or brown, and invariably with a round or rough, well-defined surface, the most common wart is called Verrucae vulgaris. This variety usually appears on the scalp, face, knees, fingers and elbows. The other common wart types include:

Genital warts: Highly contagious, these appear around the genitalia. For more information on this, see the Human Papiloma Virus section of this guide.

Pedunculated warts (skin tags): Common with advancing age, these stalk-like objects appear on the armpits, neck, scalp, chest and face.

Planters warts: Fairly common, these appear on the sole of the foot, flattened from walking.

Periungual warts: Irritation and growth usually occurs in the nail bed area.

Warts Causes

Researchers usually blame the overall incidence of warts on viruses, poor nutrition and inadequate diets, leaving the body subject to impacts by up to 35 viruses. People who rarely or never clean their bodies, a lifestyle called "poor hygiene," are sometimes more prone to get warts. Hormonal imbalances cause this condition in young adults.

While such growths are somewhat contagious, stress and advancing age sometimes emerge as contributing factors. People become more susceptible to warts as the immune system diminishes due to aging. In addition, potassium deficiencies sometimes increase the probability of getting warts. Hormonal changes during puberty often generate warts.

Wart Treatments

Homeopaths have identified and use a wide variety of natural non-toxic remedies for warts. Among the most prevalent treatments:

Diet: Changes in diet can help remove warts, particularly eating whole natural foods rather than processed meals.

Topical: Use a piece of cotton to apply solutions or oils directly on the wart, such as zinc oxide cream, castor oil, Vitamin E, Thuja oil, garlic oil, and tea tree oil.

Avoid: Never eat foods that make the body more susceptible to attack, particularly dairy products, milk, unhealthy fats, processed foods and sugar.

Sulfur: Get this vital wart-fighting mineral naturally from broccoli, cabbage, Brussels sprouts, onions and garlic.

Common remedies: Homeopaths generally prefer Graphites, Causticum, Ruta Graveolens, and Calcium carbonate.

Vitamin A: Excellent natural food sources for this essential nutrient include eggs, cold-water fish, and dark green or yellow vegetables.

Dandelion stems: These often are effective when topically applied each night and morning.

High nutrition: Enjoy foods with high or dense levels of vital nutrition such as Chlorella, maca and Spirulina.

Apple cider vinegar: Except in cases of Candida, which could be exacerbated by this substance, it's for warts as a beverage or when topically applied.

Accelerate: Speed up healing with grapefruit seed extract or lemon essential oil applied topically. These natural substances have a unpleasant taste, so immediately take a chaser after eating them.

Weight (Over)

Obesity / Overweight

Also see Waistline, Thyroid Imbalance

Rapidly increasing through epidemic proportions, being overweight or obese has been called perhaps the biggest health risk in the United States. Disturbingly, at least by some estimates a whopping 15 percent of American children suffer from obesity—a number that continues to growth. Among the entire U.S. population, an estimated 8-12 percent of all people suffer from obesity.

Rather than having what some people—rightly or wrongly—consider an "undesirable appearance," overweight people have a sharply higher risk of numerous serious and sometimes life-threatening health problems. The greatest dangers include diabetes, heart attacks, strokes and hypertension. Obese people are far more susceptible to cancers than medium-weight or thin people. Heavy individuals have a higher risk of breast, colorectal and prostate cancer.

Overweight Causes

The body mass index or BMI of some people steadily increases due to depression, which worsens as individuals get heavier. This sometimes motivates such people to take dangerous, expensive and highly addictive antidepressants that invariably take away the sex drive. The vicious spiral then continues as the person eats greater quantities of food for emotional reasons due to the loss of physical contact with others.

Perhaps the prevalent cause of overweight can be blamed on the average annual per-person consumption of sugar at 125 pounds. Besides "packing on weight," these excess sugars invariably make the body far more susceptible to a wide variety of invaders like fungi, molds, viruses and bacteria. These substances thrive on sugar, and cancer does as well. Thyroid dysfunction that leads to slow metabolisms is sometimes to blame with hypothyroidism. Menopause can be a cause.

Eating far too much food, more calories than are burned off daily, quickly or gradually leads to obesity. Any type of food when eaten in excess causes this problem, including fats, carbohydrates and proteins The gradually ballooning of body size sometimes occurs among people who fail to eat appropriate food portions, the ideal level of calories needed to correctly fuel the body.

Excess Weight and Obesity Treatments

Success in weight reduction hinges on the simultaneous use of two mutual factors, exercise and diet. Consistently burn off more calories daily than you consume while overweight, stabilizing those totals upon reaching an ideal weight. Meantime, eat moderate and sensible amounts of nutritious foods.

Some health experts recommend starting any exercise regimen with walking, careful not to begin the process at too fast a pace to avoid discouraging yourself. Weight reduction should be done gradually rather than fast by modifying the lifestyle habits of exercise and food choices. Building muscles helps burn fat; muscles require more calories than the caloric requirements of fat already within the body structure.

Avoid fruit juices that contain corn syrup, and get plenty of omega-3 fatty acids from flaxseed oil or fish oil. Exercise regularly enough to make you sweat, drinking lots of clean water to purify of any excess or loose fat. Nutrient-dense food along with proteins can help reduce or minimize hunger while preventing the body from feeling starved. Excellent foods here include bee pollen, kelp, and spinach powder, Chlorella, Spirulina and Maca.

Natural Weight Loss

Short- and long-term success in any natural weight loss program hinges on ideal nutrition. By changing or modifying food choices and lifestyle habits, one usually eliminates negative factors that cause excess weight. As an added benefit, consistent good nutrition enables the body to better fight potential disease.

Use the added bodily strength that consistent good nutrition provides over time by exercising at ideal levels—not too much and not too little.

Additionally, when consumed steadily over time good nutrition helps eliminate, lessen or minimize food cravings while eliminating unnecessary hunger. Rather than a signal that says "I'm starving to death," most instances of hunger are simply and naturally the body's way of signaling that it needs vital nutrients.

Everyone should refrain from eating too much low-nutrition food during a single sitting or continuously throughout the day. Eating this way can temporarily satisfy hunger while failing to give your body the nutrients that it actually craves. So, only eat high-nutrition, non-sugar foods in low or moderate—but not excessive—levels.

High levels of junk food forces the body to work hard to digest meals, all in a desperate attempt to find nutrients that are not there. When this happens the hunger soon returns, perhaps more intensely than shortly before, as the body continues to crave the vital nutrients that it has not been getting.

Regularly eating small portions of high-nutrition food throughout the day minimizes or eliminates hunger, while improving or maintaining optimal overall health.

Wounds

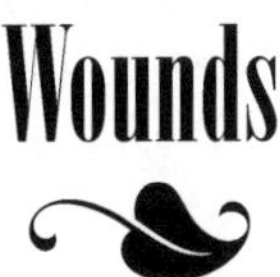

Also see Burns, Bee Stings and Insect Bites

Every wound has its own healing stage, marked by continually changing symptoms that include blood clotting, inflammation or puffiness, tingling and itching. To better understand and to address the wounds, everyone needs to know that the overall wound-healing process involves the body naturally producing capillaries and collagen needed to generate scars. The body essentially remodels itself to cover the wound and surrounding skin with protective scars.

Scarring is part of the normal healing process. But potentially severe danger sometimes erupts when infections erupt, often first marked a sense of heat, pain and spreading redness.

Wound Treatments

Prevent infection by topically applying goldenseal to the wound, taking this herb orally as well for improved results. Clean the wound or cut with immediately after the injury to prevent infection. Contrary to a popular belief that mandates using hydrogen peroxide for cleaning, refrain from using that substance which can actually damage tissue. Use plantain comprised of the pulps of aloe vera and papaya to dress wounds. Helping to prevent or minimize scars while moisturizing wounds, papaya works particularly well for bug bites and bee stings.

Accelerate healing by topically applying povidone-iodine cream, ideal as a natural antifungal, antiviral and antibacterial.

To improve overall healing, take supplements that contain beta-carotene, zinc and Vitamin C. Start clotting almost immediately by directly applying turmeric powder on bleeding cuts. Among other healing remedies and strategies:

Raw honey: This can be applied directly to wounds, excellent as an antiseptic and as an antibacterial.

Urine: Particularly when this is all that's available, this can be the only natural substance to help save a life following a serious wound. Clean, pure and antiseptic, urine contains infection-fighting antibodies.

Aggressive: Actively and aggressively treat wounds to lower leg that can lead to gangrene, particularly among diabetics who suffer injuries in that area.

Smoking: Stop smoking or avoid cigarette smoke, which ravages immunity—thereby slowing the overall healing process.

Thyroid function: People with slow metabolisms typically have slow-healing processes, so take supplements under a homeopath's guidance to boost energy.

Grape seed extract: Enables wounds to heal cleanly and quickly, while eliminating bacteria and regenerating blood vessels.

Sugar: Avoid eating this food, which can minimize immune system response by providing an environment for harmful staph to grow and to spread.

Diabetics: People with this condition should closely observe leg and feet wounds, which can be adversely affected by peripheral nerve damage.

About the Author

James W. Forsythe, M.D., H.M.D., has long been considered one of the most respected physicians in the United States, particularly for his treatment of cancer and the legal use of human growth hormone. In the mid-1960s, Dr. Forsythe graduated with honors from University of California at Berkeley and earned his medical degree from the University of California, San Francisco, before spending two years residency in Pathology at Tripler Army Hospital, Honolulu. After a tour of duty in Vietnam, he returned to San Francisco and completed an internal medicine residency and an oncology fellowship. He is also a world-renowned speaker and author. He has co-authored, been mentioned in and/or written in numerous bestselling books. To name a few: "An Alternative Medicine Definitive Guide to Cancer;" "Knockout, Interviews with Doctors who are Curing Cancer," Suzanne Somers' number one bestseller; "The Ultimate Guide to Natural Health, Quick Reference A-Z Directory of Natural Remedies for Diseases and Ailments;" "Anti-Aging Cures;" "The Healing Power of Sleep;" "Anti-Aging Sleep Secrets;" "Outsmart Your Cancer: Alternative Non-Toxic Treatments That Work;" and "Compassionate Oncology—What Conventional Cancer Specialists Don't Want You To Know;" and "Obaminable Care," "Complete Pain;" "Natural Painkillers;" and "Your Secret to the Fountain of Youth—What They Don't Want You to Know About HGH Human Growth Hormone;" "Take Control of Your Cancer;" "Emergency Radiation Medical Handbook," and the "About Death From a Cancer Doctor's Perspective."

Contact Information
Century Wellness Clinic
521 Hammill Lane
Reno, NV, 89511
(775) 827-0707
RenoWellnessDr@Yahoo.com
DrForsythe.com

TRUE DIRECTIONS

An affiliate of Tarcher Books

OUR MISSION

Tarcher's mission has always been to publish books that contain great ideas. Why? Because:

GREAT LIVES BEGIN WITH GREAT IDEAS

At Tarcher, we recognize that many talented authors, speakers, educators, and thought-leaders share this mission and deserve to be published – many more than Tarcher can reasonably publish ourselves. True Directions is ideal for authors and books that increase awareness, raise consciousness, and inspire others to live their ideals and passions.

Like Tarcher, True Directions books are designed to do three things: inspire, inform, and motivate.

Thus, True Directions is an ideal way for these important voices to bring their messages of hope, healing, and help to the world.

Every book published by True Directions– whether it is non-fiction, memoir, novel, poetry or children's book – continues Tarcher's mission to publish works that bring positive change in the world. We invite you to join our mission.

For more information, see the True Directions website:
www.iUniverse.com/TrueDirections/SignUp

Be a part of Tarcher's community to bring positive change in this world! See exclusive author videos, discover new and exciting books, learn about upcoming events, connect with author blogs and websites, and more!
www.tarcherbooks.com

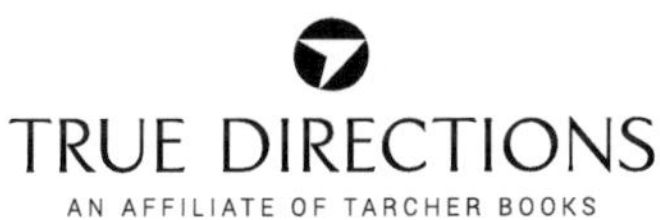